"The last twenty years have brought us marvelous new insights, skills, and discoveries about intimate, loving sex. Charla has succeeded in distilling them into a form that's easy to read, easy to follow, and easy to do—for just about anyone. This book will save you trudging through fifteen others, looking for the gems."

—Betty Martin, D.C., Intimacy Coach and founder of The Institute for Erotic Education

"Charla Hathaway shows herself to be masterful at presenting some exquisitely helpful ideas for heterosexual couples wishing to improve their erotic and loving connection. This is a truly beautiful book."

—Barnaby B. Barratt, Ph.D., D.H.S., Director of the Center for Tantric Spirituality

"*Eight Erotic Nights* delivers deep, intimate teachings in a sexy and playful way that is easy to understand and share. Whether it's cuddling innocently on the couch or canoodling lustily between the sheets, this book and its valuable practices will give you amazing tools to achieve a lifetime of heightened pleasure!"

—Reid Mihalko, sex and relationship educator and creator of Cuddle Party (cuddleparty.com)

"With enthusiastic candor, Charla Hathaway cheerfully guides readers through a sensually seductive adventure to discover their erotic potential."

—Karen Kreps, author of *Intimacies: Secrets of Love, Sex & Romance*

For Mary & Jim

Journey into the heart & soul
of your loving & enjoy
each breath, each sigh

Chaka Khan

2011

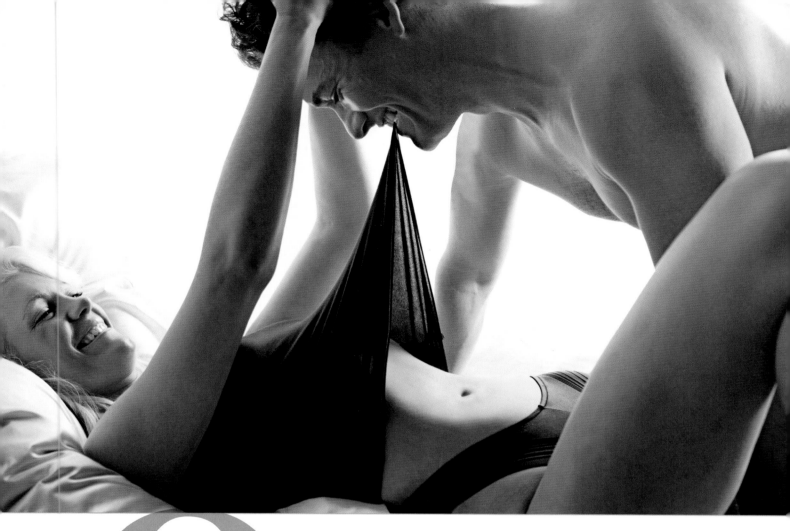

8 Erotic Nights

Passionate Encounters That Inspire Great Sex for a Lifetime

CHARLA HATHAWAY
AUTHOR OF *EROTIC MASSAGE*

QUIVER

First published in the USA in 2008 by
Quiver, a member of
Quayside Publishing Group
100 Cummings Center
Suite 406-L
Beverly, MA 01915-6101
www.quiverbooks.com

The publisher maintains the records relating to images in this book required by
18 USC 2257. Records are located at Rockport Publishers, Inc., 100 Cummings
Center, Suite 406-L, Beverly, MA 01915-6101.

12 11 10 09 08 1 2 3 4 5

ISBN-13: 978-1-59233-310-3
ISBN-10: 1-59233-310-9

Library of Congress Cataloging-in-Publication Data

Hathaway, Charla.
  Eight erotic nights: passionate encounters that inspire great sex for a lifetime /
Charla Hathaway.
     p. cm.
  ISBN 1-59233-310-9
  1. Sex instruction. 2. Sex. 3. Sexual excitement. I. Title.
  HQ31.H384 2008
  613.9'6--dc22
                          2007040878

Cover design: Carol Holtz
Photography: Thomas Anders
Author photo: Wade H.B. Matthews, Jr.

Printed and bound in Singapore

For all couples seeking greater truth and trust to
strengthen their sexual connection.

CONTENTS

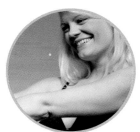
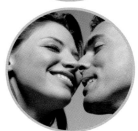
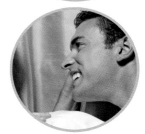
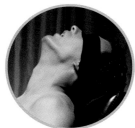
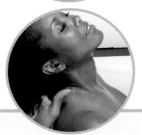

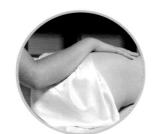
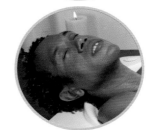
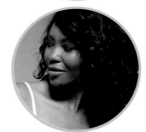
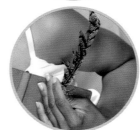
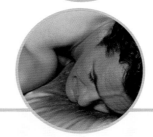

INTRODUCTION

Eight Erotic Nights is a guidebook for couples who desire to expand their erotic potential. What is erotic sex? It's sex that enables you to experience more sensation in your body, connect more passionately with your partner, deepen your orgasms, and reclaim a sense of discovery about your lovemaking. It's sex for the soul as well as the body.

Eight Erotic Nights is a sequential series of sensual activities that will help you build a foundation of truth and trust with your partner and deepen sexual excitement. The eight-minute Daily Erotic Ritual, for example, teaches you simple ways to leave the day behind, chart a new direction, and drop into expansive body time. This daily joyful exercise hones your erotic skills and lays the foundation for your Erotic Nights.

Each evening of delightful play is skillfully designed to take you step by step into the joyful heart of your sexuality. You will reignite sexual rapture by experiencing surprise, uncertainty, awe, and compassion with your partner. Breath by breath, touch by touch, and night after night, you will renew your relationship with yourself and your partner, awakening the erotic and nourishing your soul.

Each night session starts by reflecting back to material covered in the last session and ends with a looking ahead exercise (which will take you about twenty minutes to complete) to prepare you for the next night's adventure. You'll want to read each night/chapter ahead of that evening's erotic encounter.

Every turn-on in *Eight Erotic Nights* is about individual choice and honoring each other's uniqueness. Some exercises may require you and your partner to be emotionally vulnerable. Thus, each evening is finely constructed with a backdrop of safety and confidentiality so that you feel free to discover and grow. Remember: Feeling safe comes before feeling sexy. You are encouraged to check in with yourself, not simply mirror your partner, and to be motivated by your own desires and pleasure.

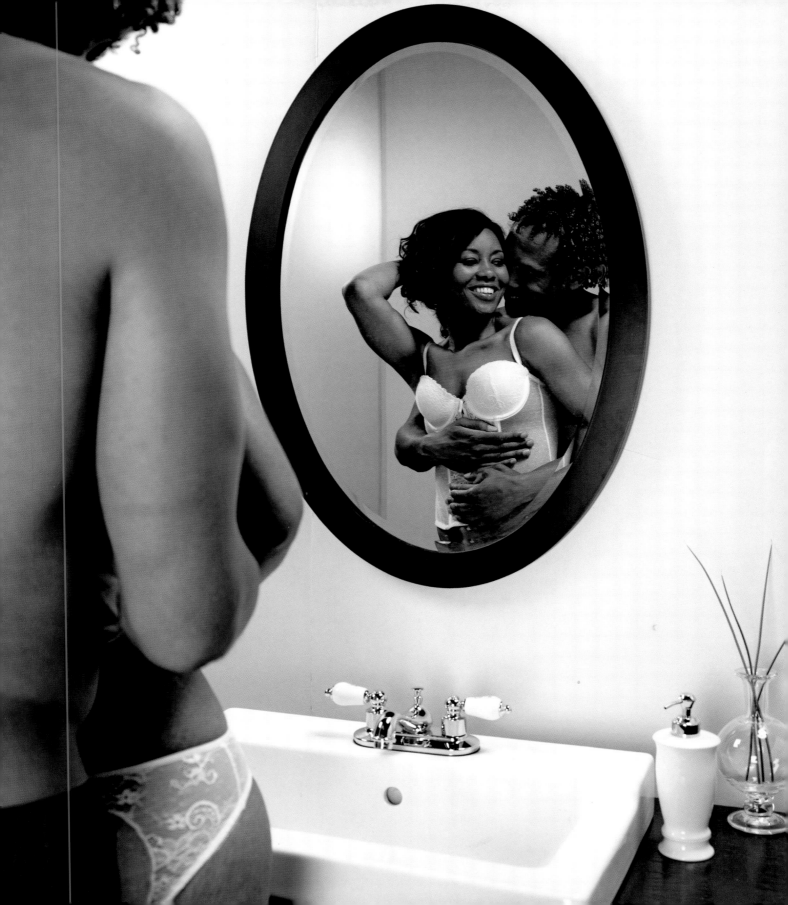

You may decide to schedule your Erotic Nights once a week, which will make your total journey last for two months. Or you may only choose to commit to once a month. My recommendation for continuity and momentum is to schedule Erotic Nights two times a month, like the first and third Wednesday (or a weekend night), in which case you would complete the whole book in four months.

Eight Erotic Nights starts with putting pleasure at the top of your agenda and committing to experiencing fun in your life. You'll then learn, with your partner, to develop focused attention that feels divine to give and receive. You'll practice saying yes and no only when you mean it and learn how to Come Clean with your partner by releasing withheld emotions. You'll learn to recognize your desires as your highest intelligence, and rather than being shamed by them, you will embrace and express them.

This book also offers you tools and rituals for showing approval and appreciation for your partner's body. You'll learn to experience and appreciate each other, rather than control and judge. You'll give up pretending and working at sex (which only dulls your sensations and appetite) and start doing only what brings you pleasure in the moment. This book is your simple and profound map to erotic wellness, wisdom, and freedom.

Often, sex is boring because we get into routines simply out of lack of attention and the failure to see what is possible. So each Erotic Night has delicious, sensuous body touching exercises to electrify your erotic imagination and fuel your desires. Most of us have not explored the positive power of our sexual shadows or empowered our sexuality by inviting our "inner opposite gender" to come out and play. Watch the fireworks when his inner female is being seduced, stoked, and taken care of by her inner male.

In this book, I provide a good look at relationship models and discuss how to make conscious and changeable agreements that address erotic and sexual needs. As you and your partner build a foundation of truth and trust, you will be empowered to reveal—instead of conceal—your true sexual desires and enliven your relationship with honesty. Many sexual challenges, such as the frequency and type of touch, can be lovingly and creatively addressed in consensual agreements.

You do not need a soul mate, a spouse, or even a lifetime partner for a successful journey through *Eight Erotic Nights.* All you need is a commitment from a good friend to explore with you the activities of this book over an agreed-upon time frame, secured by the promise of confidentiality. Both of you will enrich and nourish your future relationships by practicing the book's exercises together.

The erotic encounters in this book are more sensual than sexual in nature. Most exercises can be done with clothes on if preferred. Each of the eight Erotic Nights develops the lost art of cultivating and containing sexual juice in greater and greater quantities until it spills over to everything you do. Withholding sexual energy is an ancient art lost in today's world of "get it now." On Erotic Nights, I recommend savoring one another, building desire, and not dissipating the sexual charge through orgasmic release. I suggest a commitment at the beginning to save intercourse or penetration sex for another night. The exercises you do in this book will only enrich your capacity to experience pleasure.

You probably grew up in a family and community that did not know how to nurture your innate sexual curiosity and play. No one gave you a model for cultivating great sex; instead you may have encountered silence, shame, and mixed messages. Isn't it time you take the lead and plan a pleasureable path for your precious partnership?

Sex is natural. If you've been brought up to think otherwise, you've been lied to. And there is no right way to do it. There's just your way, in this moment, with this person, and with this guidebook. *Eight Erotic Nights* will take you back to your authentic, joyous erotic being.

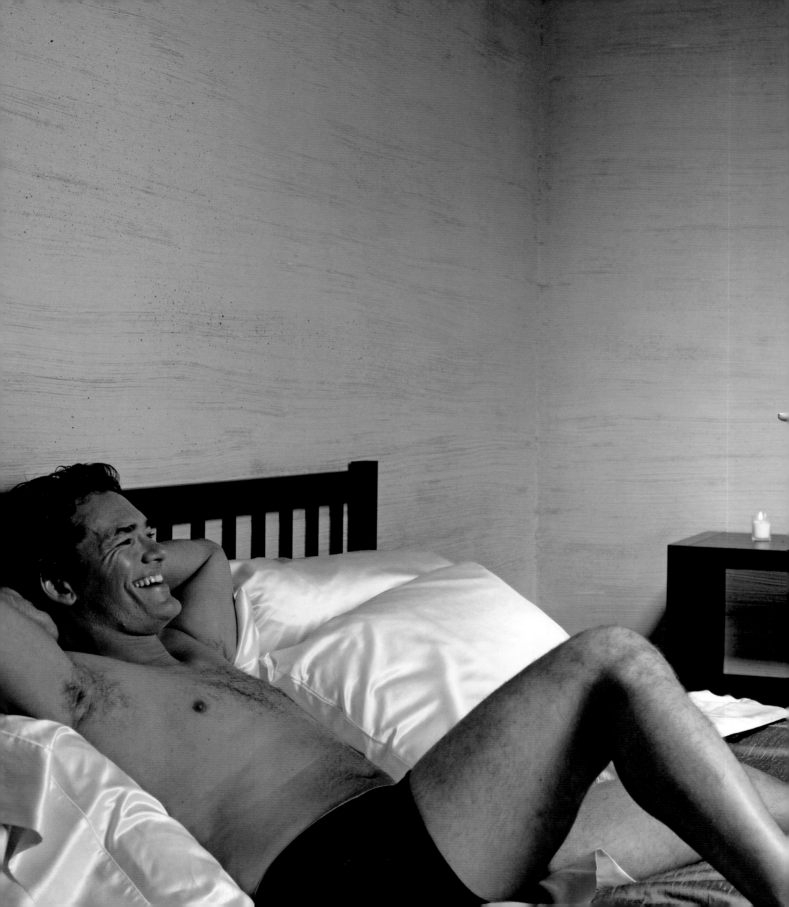

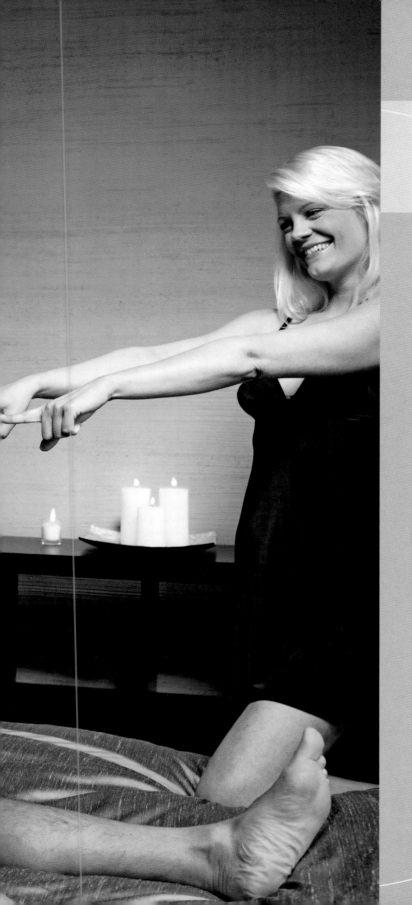

YOUR JOYRIDE TO GREAT SEX

Becoming a Pleasure Activist

YOUR JOYRIDE TO GREAT SEX:
BECOMING A PLEASURE ACTIVIST

Are you ready to expand your capacity for erotic enjoyment? Are you ready to experience a more loving connection with your partner? Are you ready to have great sex for a lifetime? Well hang on, because your life is about to take a sharp turn. This ride is not about the status quo, and here's the disclaimer you need to know: You may find yourself suspended in prolonged orgasmic realms and erotic trance states. This rapturous experience will likely spill over onto other parts of your life in strange and wonderful ways such as loving yourself, your body, and others with renewed ease and zest. You may approve and appreciate your partner like never before. That said, welcome to a journey straight into a sacred and erotic way of being in your body.

You are about to get serious about having fun. When you have fun with your partner, your love grows; when the fun stops, your relationship withers. When you're having fun, girlfriend, you don't need to be rescued by a guy. When you're having fun, gentleman, you don't need to "give" her an orgasm or be responsible for her happiness. Whew! You can begin to settle back into this newfound space, breathe deeply, and allow yourself to simply feel your own feelings. By tuning into your sensations, you become free to feel the subtle shades of your own arousal and pleasure.

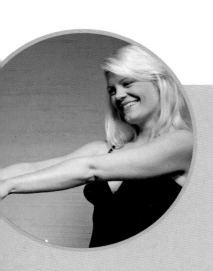

Coming from Joy

Do what brings you joy. No payback, obligation, manipulation, or pretending during sex. Only do something because it turns *you* on. Fill up your own cup, and when it overflows it will spill out onto your partner. You need to become your own wonder-generating machine, because if you don't, you'll be sucking it out of another. So be the seeker, not the sucker, and generate your own awe and wonder for each moment you live.

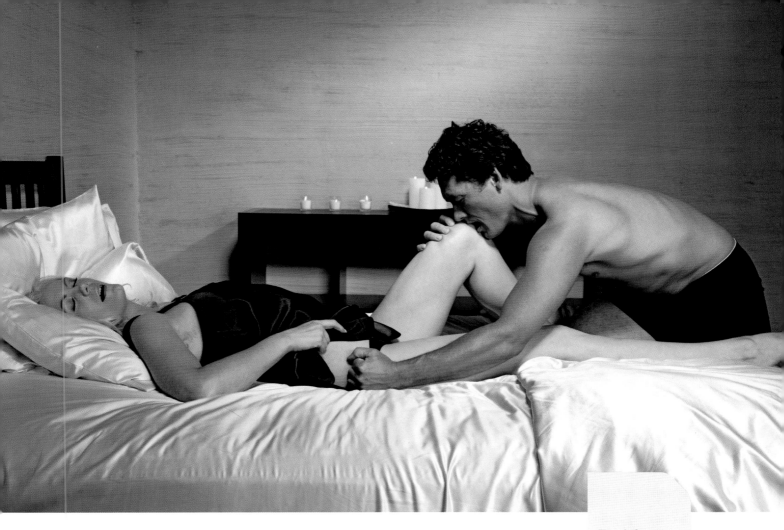

Touch for *your* pleasure. Touch to turn yourself on.

Now this isn't the message you grew up with, especially when it came to sex. You learned that sex is all about pleasing or "doing" the other person. And in trying so hard to "do" her or him, you've been getting wrapped up in performing, which separates you from the joy of the moment, makes you anxious, and causes you to worry about not doing it right.

You may become so involved in trying to turn on the other person that you forget to turn yourself on. Sex becomes about "doing," and you leave your bodies and get into your heads. If you are trying to please your partner, you are performing, and your partner will feel the subtle pressure to reassure you that you're doing a great job—no matter what is really happening in his or her body. Neither you nor your partner is free to feel true sensations.

Instead of performing on each other, do what's right for you in the moment with an agreement that if it doesn't feel good to your partner, she will tell you. Her body becomes a playground for you to explore for your pleasure. You'll be more inclined to surrender into gorgeous altered states of ecstasy when you don't have to take care of your partner. You'll learn to trust that taking care of yourself is the best way to take care of another.

Understanding Pleasure

Most of us have a knee-jerk reaction to showing up for pleasure. In my case, the new man in my life lived far away. After a wonderful visit together, he suggested that we do the cross-country drive back together, instead of me driving home alone. He wanted us to camp next to his favorite waterfall, watch the meteorite showers, and check out a couple of secluded hot springs along the way. He said he would go with me halfway home, then take a train back and send me on my way. I gasped at the thought of such wonder and almost perfunctorily said no. There's a fear and uncertainty about claiming wonder. I was ready to utter some excuse about getting home early enough, but stopped myself, looked him straight in the eye, and said a solid "yes." It was four days of heaven in my life.

You may not experience pleasure well because it's so different from how you're conditioned to experience life. You're afraid of what to do with it. You fear stepping out of your old habits. It's more comfortable to recount stories of lack, disappointment, and hardship than it is to share your successes and joy. Well, I say no more bonding in the woe-is-me mode. Let's instead start bonding over the positive—by flirting and bragging about our successes.

BECOME A PLEASURE ACTIVIST

Becoming a Pleasure Activist gives you—and others around you—permission to experience more pleasure. Your parents didn't likely tell you how important pleasure is to bonding partnerships or families. Your schools pitted you against one another and piled on the work. Your churches extolled sacrifice and delayed gratification. And the workplace wants to handcuff you to achievement.

What if you decide instead to handcuff yourself to your desires? What if you start to embrace desires instead of being afraid or ashamed of them? What if you believe your desires are your deepest wisdom and highest intelligence? What abundance and pleasure would you create by freely claiming and expressing heartfelt longings? While reading *Eight Erotic Nights,* you will give into your desires and allow them to guide your play with joy.

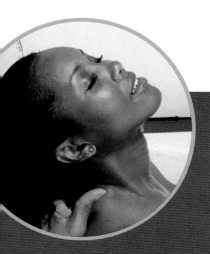

"I was amazed at how **doing only what brought me joy** made loving my partner so juicy for both of us. Before, I was so busy trying to please him I didn't even feel my own arousal.

THE PLEASURE BRAIN

Pleasure is about lessening the grip of the controlling, judging, and evaluating mind and inviting the "other mind" to come forth. Your other mind (or right brain) has a different wisdom. This intelligence longs to know life through experiencing the mystery, welcoming uncertainty, being present in the moment, and relishing sensual pleasure in the body.

This gracious wisdom is the fuel for your journey back to your erotic being. When you are aware of bodily sensations, you are in this "other way of being." Your body knows only the present moment, unencumbered by the past and future. Innate body wisdom invites you to feel, to be, and to surrender yourself to the moment.

I used to think being a good lover was about what I did in bed—how I could make my partner feel. In my maturity, I now know that being a good lover isn't about "doing" at all. Rather, it is summed up in a series of questions: How much can I let go? How much can I surrender in this moment? How much can I receive, feel the sensations in my body, melt into a caress, and witness the wonder of life reflected in my lover's gaze? Become a Pleasure Activist, and surrender is just around the next bend. Slide over, baby, we're on our way.

Start Flirting:
Attention without Intention

Try flirting to find your turned-on, sassy self. What's more, do it often—with old men at the bus stop, the dork at work, the butcher, the woman carrying groceries, or just about anybody. Flirt because you can, and because you know how it makes you feel. Flirt because it's a joy to give away your sparkle, which seems to come back bigger each time you give it away. You'll learn who is in charge of your turn-on and who gets your juices running . . . you!

When I stopped trying to do it 'right' for him and did what was right for me in the moment, **I felt so turned on.** It freed him up to feel his own feelings too without needing to reassure me."

—YVONNE, AGE 27

Scheduling Pleasure: Great Sex Is a Discipline

If great sex is where you choose to go, you're going to have to carve out the time to practice it—a few minutes every day and at least eight evenings over the next months. Scheduling and committing to pleasure is just like anything else you want to accomplish in your life. If you want to get good at something, you make time for it; you put it on the agenda.

Think of the things you do well in your life. Maybe it is your job, raising a family, playing golf, dancing, or whatever. Look at the time you have spent becoming good at it. Look at the years you studied, trained, went to school, and practiced, and think of how many teachers helped you. We spend more time getting good at our careers than studying and practicing our relationships.

If fine-tuning a sensual relationship is on your agenda, sit down with your partner and make a clear agreement as to how you will use this book. First of all, you both need to commit to the journey. If one partner is reluctant, you may start by committing to just a segment of the journey and then reevaluating as you go. Ideally, you are both willing to commit to five Daily Erotic Rituals (each eight minutes) a week and eight (two- to three-hour) Erotic Nights over two to eight months. You can revise your agreement at any time by telling your partner. Doing everything this book suggests will take approximately thirty-two hours of your life. In fewer hours than a work week, your relationship (and life!) will be sexually transformed. How you make love will be forever changed.

Second, discuss how much time each week you will commit to daily partnered exercise and the best time of the day for the both of you. You'll begin to look forward to this few-minute ritual as a way to relax and connect in "body time." You can even do this ritual over the phone. Good times for the Daily Erotic Ritual are when you arrive home from work, before dinner, or before bed. Choose a time, and be consistent.

Next, decide what frequency of Erotic Nights fits both of your schedules. It could be once a week, once every other week, or once a month. Pick an evening of the week—any one will do—and agree to a specific three-hour time frame for that evening. Write all eight

Banish "Should"

Stop "shoulding" all over yourself. Don't just do something, stand there! Slow down, go nowhere, do nothing, meander without direction, and even get a little lost—for these are the qualities that make sex great. They delight us in the bedroom and turn us into curious children captured on the edge of discovery. If you're trying to get somewhere, you aren't there.

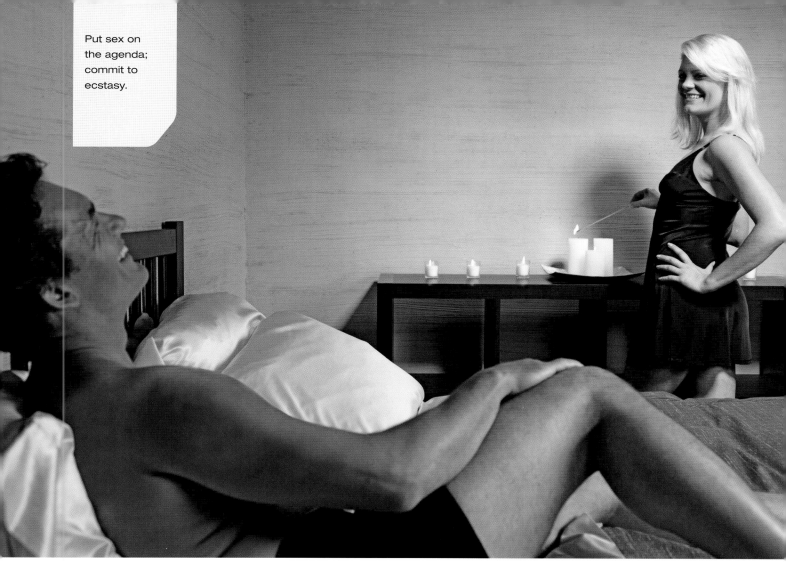

Put sex on the agenda; commit to ecstasy.

dates into both of your calendars spanning ahead two, four, or eight months. Agree that these dates are to be treated with the same respect (or more) as any other date on your calendar, be it business, recreational, or family.

In Preparation: Keeping an Ecstasy Journal

You and your partner each need a small notebook, which will be your Ecstasy Journal. Start by writing in your journal the three commitments you have just made in scheduling your pleasure. Your entries may look similar to the examples below:

MY COMMITMENTS TO PLEASURE
Commitment #1: "I commit to <u>five</u> (eight-minute) Daily Erotic Rituals a week together with my partner <u>before dinner</u>."

Commitment #2: "I commit to eight Erotic Nights with my partner, meeting <u>the first and third Saturdays of the month</u>, starting date <u>January 12 from 7 p.m. to 10 p.m.</u>

Commitment #3: "I commit to this schedule for pleasure with the same respect and integrity I assign other commitments. I will notify my partner in advance of any revisions to the above schedule or change in my commitments to the erotic journey together."

Sign and date this journal entry. Bravo! You've just accomplished the nuts and bolts of great sex. You're on your way.

In Preparation: Creating a Sensual Space for Erotic Encounters

Take a look at the space where you plan to spend your nights of erotic exploration. Does this room exude a warmth and sensuality that encourage you to unveil your passion, expose your vulnerable self, and languish in playful encounters with a partner? This outer environment can be a reflection of your inward journey. Make it soft, plush, rich, and sexy.

Before your first Erotic Night, make whatever preparations you feel will enhance the beauty of your surroundings. Each partner can take responsibility to add several things of his or her choosing to dress up the room and transform it into an erotic enclave for adventures.

You may choose a few candles, an array of peacock feathers for the night stand, soft fabric to cover the blinds, or a sheepskin or soft rug for the floor. Soft lighting, soothing music (without lyrics), a silk scarf, scented lotions, a rabbit fur mitt, and extra pillows add to the ambiance. Just a string of well-placed, small Christmas tree lights in a large plant or softly hanging in front of fabric can transform the feel of a room. Erotic art for the wall and a well-placed mirror or two can add excitement.

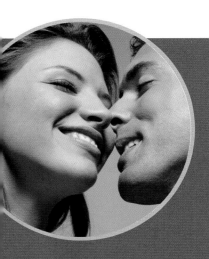

"My boyfriend called me up at work and invited me to **a special night of loving**—a whole week ahead of time! On that night, after a pampering bath and erotic story, he carried me into his bedroom—**what a surprise!** He'd dressed up the bed in satin sheets and soft silk pillows,

Commit to several ways in which you will contribute to the Sensual Space for your erotic exploring, and write them down in your Ecstasy Journal. Delight in your own unique taste and personal touches when choosing and shopping. Write on your calendar when you will add or install your contributions, and make it several days before the first Erotic Night so you will not feel rushed for your first date. Your new environs will hold your passion, and just passing by the door will make you smile.

In Preparation: Readying Your Mind and Body

On the day of your Erotic Night, drink lots of water, get some exercise, and pay special attention to your diet. Eat lightly and choose foods that digest easily, like vegetables and fruits, to enhance your mind's attention and body's sensations. If you are inspired, buy a gift for your beloved, show up with a rose, or write an appreciative card. You will be setting the stage for the wonder to unfold.

The evening of your date night, refrain from coffee or alcohol, except perhaps a single glass of wine if desired. Shower or treat yourself to a luxurious bath. Prepare your mouth with special attention for the close breathing exercises that, with a fresh breath, can be a divine exchange of essences. Breathing with and into each other is a delicious suspension of our usual awareness.

Now, be punctual; start and end your Erotic Night on time. Arrive with an open mind and a soft heart, leaving your expectations and knowledge at the door. Take time to settle into your body with a few deep breaths and remember that you have everything you need to experience joy. Don't be rushed in your preparation for the evening. Be kind to yourself, and schedule some down-time before and after each session.

hung erotic art—including naked pictures of us—on the walls, and arranged on the bed stand candles, lotions, and feathers. **I gazed astounded through watery eyes at the sacred temple he had created for us."**

—BERYL, AGE 49

Slowing Down to the Speed of Love

Just how much of your surroundings do you notice when you're racing down the inter-state at seventy-five miles per hour versus meandering down a winding country road on a Sunday afternoon? Sometimes we don't know how to shift out of high gear. We're so busy "doing" that we've forgotten how to quit.

The art of slowness is not valued in our culture. It's typical to keep heaping more "shoulds" on your plate and measure your self-worth by crossing things off a list. Relationships, especially intimate ones, are the axis of learning in life, yet you may toss them only the crumbs of energy left over from your hectic days.

Erotic Exercise 1: Consciously Connecting through the Daily Erotic Ritual [EIGHT MINUTES]

Just eight minutes is enough to change gears, slow down, leave the day behind, and ease into a spacious, erotic way of being with your partner. You will learn to "clear" with one another about your day (two minutes each; four minutes total), set intention (one minute), and Ocean Breathe together (three minutes). This short ritual will open your heart, focus your mind, and relax your body—which is where you want to be for erotic play. It will prime your success in unforeseen ways for longer erotic evenings. In this daily discipline, you flex the muscle of conscious connection and sacred embodiment that lays the foundation for luscious Erotic Nights.

By now you've already decided what time of day works best for you both to begin this exercise. Keep a timer on hand—it will be used for many of the exercises in this book—and commit to keeping strict time frames for the exercise. Staying within the time frames will solidify your commitment to the ritual and keep interest high. If you extend beyond the time frame, you will miss the power of the exercise. This may lead you to decide the ritual

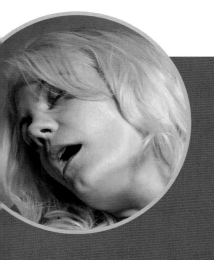

"After days of taking just a minute to speak our releases and intentions, I realize how **letting go of stuff** created the space for us to shape the rest of the evening into a more positive, self-loving interaction. I've adopted this ritual in other

doesn't work and to drop it. Honoring time frames not only makes this ritual pivotal but also paves the way for cherishable Erotic Nights.

1. **Find a quiet place to sit together** with knees touching or in a loose yab-yum position (legs lapped over each other), as illustrated on page 25.

2. **Loosen your clothing,** especially around the waist, and kick off your shoes. Make yourself as comfortable as possible.

3. **Decide who will share first**—perhaps the person who needs it the most. Make sure you alternate from time to time. Agree with your partner that what is said in Sensual Space stays there. Ensuring a mutual commitment to confidentiality provides the safety you need to speak freely.

Now connect with the following exercises.

WEATHER REPORTING: BE SEEN AND HEARD (FOUR MINUTES)

Often there is something we need to get off our chests before we can settle comfortably into our bodies and share an intimate space with another. Until it's out, we can't think of anything else. This two-minute "clearing" allows you to vent about the most pressing issues or frustrations (without going on too long about them) so that you can become more present with your partner. Getting present through the Weather Report is like a relationship tune-up: It paves the way for a smooth ride into feeling close and sexy with your partner.

Set the timer for two minutes. Using weather terminology, the first person begins to describe his day or emotional state. He may say things such as, "It feels sunny at work; my proposal is garnering the attention it deserves, and it's growing in promise . . ." Or, "My day was partly cloudy, and I'm afraid a cool fog is creeping in." The speaker may choose to talk about his day, work, kids, relationships, etc.

places, too, like at work, because **it is so powerful to change a negative direction into a positive experience.** I see how setting intention helps me create my feelings, moment by moment."

—MARSHA, AGE 32

The first speaker talks for the full two minutes without interruption, unless the listener needs to ask a quick, clarifying question to understand a point. The listener does not offer feedback, evaluate, add his or her experience, or even offer encouragement. The listener, with focused attention, simply takes in or hears what the speaker is saying.

After the two-minute timer sounds, wind off your last sentence, take a couple of deep breaths together, reset the timer, and switch roles. Refrain from speaking between roles. As the second speaker, resist any inclination to "mirror" the tone of the first speaker; come from your own experience even if your outlook is sunny while your partner is getting rained on.

Because you may not feel anyone truly listens to you in your life, or you may not have developed strong listening skills, the Weather Report is a validating and precious gift you can give each other. You'll learn to listen from the heart without needing to solve or advise your partner. Rather, you'll spend quality time simply "being" with your partner and holding space for you both to embrace your feelings.

RELEASE AND SET INTENTION (ONE MINUTE)

Learning to release what no longer serves you and to call in by name that which you desire is a powerful way to focus the mind for change. By first clearing out what is not working for you and then putting attention to what you desire, you'll dissipate what you don't want and attract what you do want. The mere voicing of a release and intention spins the cosmic wheels in a magical way. Setting intention before sex transforms it from mundane into sacred and empowers the encounter with consciousness.

After sharing Weather Reports, take turns of thirty seconds each to offer something you are ready to let go of in the moment and something you intentionally call into your life. Offer to release anything that you wish to decrease. Use one short sentence, such as, "I release the anger I felt today when my boss told me to redo the project." Or, "I release my anxiety

Weather Report Review

You may want later to revisit with your partner something brought up during the Weather Report. This is a natural response to heartfelt exchanges. Respectfully ask your partner for permission at the later time to revisit a topic brought up in your Sensual Space. You may say something like, "I would like to hear more about such and such that you brought up in your Weather Report. Would you be willing to talk more about it?" Your Sensual Space will open you in vulnerable and sensitive ways, so do not assume you can go charging in later on the same note, or the fragile container of trust will be broken.

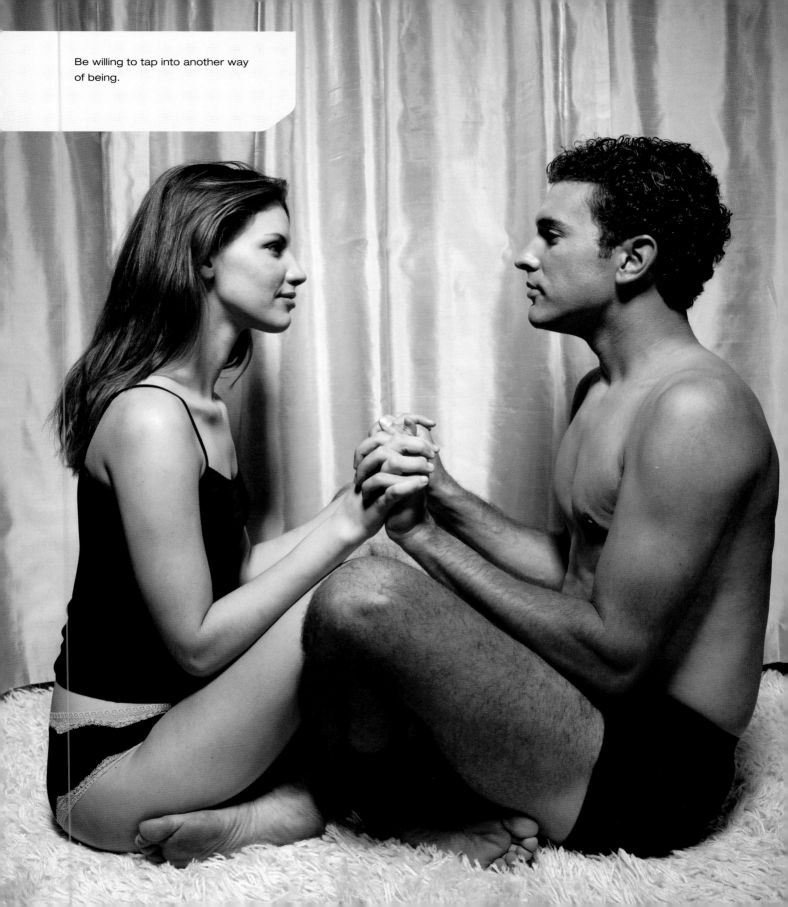

Be willing to tap into another way of being.

over not having finished writing the second chapter." By releasing stress, worry, and tension from the day, you transition into a more sensual, sexy, and peaceful place.

Follow your release with your intention, spoken in a short, positive affirmation, such as, "I intend to open my heart to appreciate my family," or "I intend to feel good about doing nothing for a while." Voice your intention in positive language. For example, if you don't want to feel sef-doubt, you may say, "I intend to feel loved by myself and others tonight."

SOUL GAZE AND OCEAN BREATHE (THREE MINUTES)

Breathing slowly and deeply together so you can hear the sound of the ocean in your breath is a delicious and restful ritual for slowing down. Awareness to your breath rids the mind of chatter and moves erotic energy through the whole body. Conscious breathing is your ticket to feeling more sensation in the body and prolonging blissful states of erotic trance. And your daily practice of erotic breathing techniques will prepare you for moving erotic energy generated in one area, say, the genitals, into electrifying, whole-body experiences during Erotic Nights.

Sit across from your partner cross-legged with your knees touching, or sit on your partner's lap. Set the timer for three minutes, but remember, this is not a time to watch the clock. Look into the left eye of your partner with a soft gaze. Be aware of the space behind each other's eyes. Gently gaze into the "window of the soul" of your beloved and see your divine nature being reflected back to you through your partner's eyes. In Tantra, the ancient practice of sacred loving, this is called Soul Gazing.

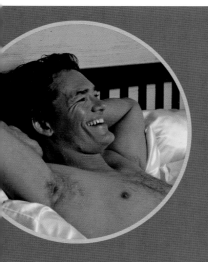

"Ocean Breathing with my partner gets me **into my body and out of my head**—just the place I want to go more in sex. Often three minutes seems too short, and we improvise. **Consistent practice has made the longer night exercises easier and really hot."**

—IRWIN, AGE 34

While Soul Gazing, allow your attention to go completely to your breath. Practice Ocean Breathing by constricting your nostrils slightly on the inhale so you can hear the air stream coming in through your nose. Remember when you were a child and someone put a shell up to your ear and said, "Listen, can you hear the ocean inside?" That's the sound you want to make through your nose with each inhale. Now let your belly go soft, and let your mind follow the ocean sound of your breath all the way into your belly.

On the exhale, open your mouth slightly, and let out an "aaaahh" as if you were fogging up a mirror with your moist, warm breath. Soften your throat, and feel the vibrations as you sigh or moan on the exhale. Let the sound flow out effortlessly through your open throat. Sense how joyful it is to rest all of your attention on this most natural of all movements, the flow of the breath.

Learn to "ride the sound" of each breath by following the air coming in and falling out of the body. Yogis know that if you can follow your breath you are in the present moment. Meditative and spiritual sexuality practices such as Tantra (the yoga of sex) start with awareness of the breath. Direct your mind, over and over again, to follow the sound of each breath.

Notice your partner's breath. Is it slower or faster than yours? Listen for your partner's breath. Can you hear each other? Take a deep breath in, and let out a huge vibrating "aaaaaah" together on the exhale. Go ahead and laugh at yourselves, two human vibrators resonating as one. Making sounds cultivates a juicier flow of erotic energy and shakes loose the old inhibitions of the body. No wonder we were told to be quiet when we breathe.

You may naturally find a rhythm between you and begin synchronizing your breathing. You may begin to notice a suspension of ordinary time and reality; just follow the sound of the breath in and out. Resist the temptation to feel silly and the need to return to the familiar; you're on the edge of a delicious and soothing trance. You can assure the thinking mind that you will return after a few minutes of observing your breath.

Be willing to tap into another way of being. Your sense of separateness melts, self-doubt evaporates, and you feel energized and relaxed at the same time. Focused breath becomes the pathway to connection with your partner and the whole cosmos. Long practiced by the mystics of many traditions, this awareness of the breath has been overlooked by us in the West. Yet awareness of the breath is a simple, profound tool for personal transformation. Meditative and spiritual sexuality practices such as Tantra start with awareness of the breath.

Enjoy the permission to gaze upon your beloved, share the same breath, and make sounds together. Observe how a softness falls over your partner's face. When your mind wanders off on a thought, catch it, and gently return your attention to the sound of the breath. This exercise can feel like coming home to yourself—or even like making gentle love to your partner.

End the ritual of Ocean Breathing with a Heart Salutation. Place your hands together in prayer position at your heart, your thumbs touching your breast bone. Take a deep breath with your partner, lean forward in a bow toward each other, and exhale. A Heart Salutation honors the divine spark inherent in each of us. It brings closure to the many activities you'll be practicing in this book with a clean sense of separation.

Looking Ahead

Congratulations! You have accomplished the nuts and bolts of great sex by scheduling time for pleasure both in Daily Erotic Rituals and Erotic Nights. You've written these dates and times into your calendar and Ecstasy Journal. You've read how to do the Daily Erotic Ritual with Weather Reports, Setting Intentions, and Ocean Breathing together. You've agreed to practice the ritual a certain number of times.

You've also committed to preparing a sensual space for erotic play, as well as your mind and body, before your first Erotic Night. Think about it: You tune up your car for high performance, and now you're going to tune up your sex life. On your first night, you'll feast on the food of love, revel in undivided attention, and add new tools to your rapturous toolbox!

Read Erotic Night One several days before it takes place.

Erotic Recap

- Scheduling Pleasure
- In Preparation: Keeping an Ecstasy Journal
- In Preparation: Creating a Sensual Space for Erotic Encounters
- In Preparation: Readying Your Mind and Body
- Consciously Connecting through the Daily Erotic Ritual: *eight minutes*

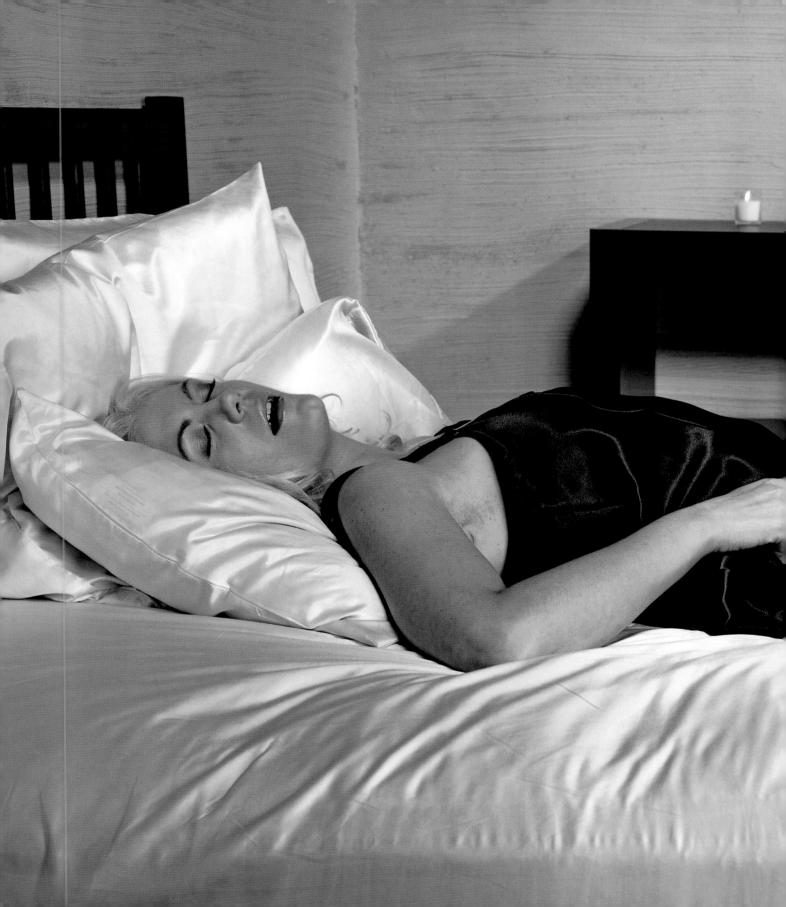

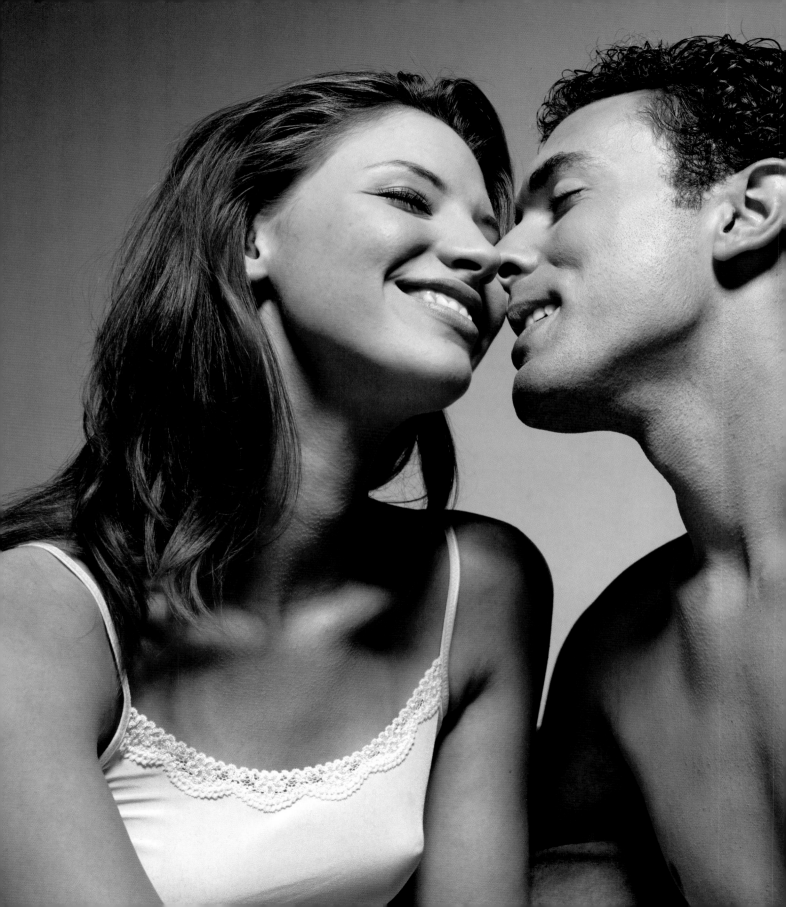

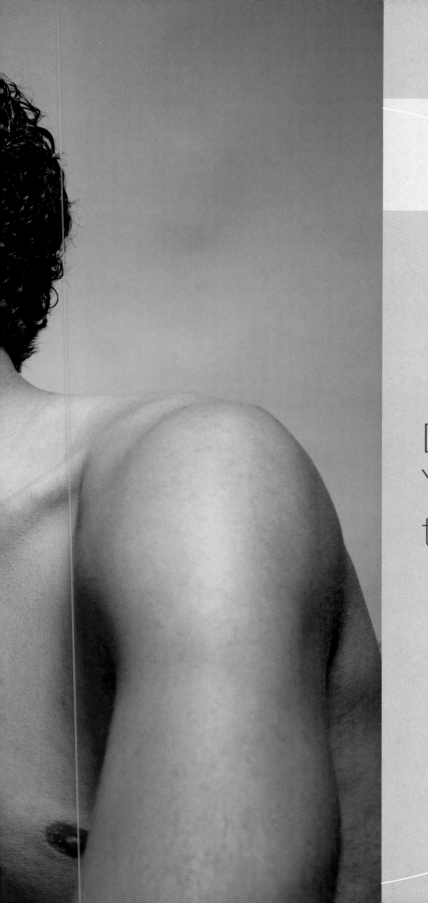

EROTIC NIGHT
ONE

Deepening
Your Attention
to Love

EROTIC NIGHT
ONE

Love is either growing or dying; it is not static. In long-term relationships, we often stop noticing the other person, begin to assume things about our partner, and generally take the relationship for granted. The excitement of new love—the initial Free Trial Offer—expires, and our attention wanes.

Over time in relationships, you may feel more afraid to take risks or "rock the boat" than you did in the beginning. You may opt to protect your partner's feelings and play it safe to protect your long-term "investment." However, this doesn't make for great sex. After spending time not getting what you want, you'll feel resentful; you'll become tense and numbed in the pelvic region. Many couples eventually give up on sex.

During your first Erotic Night, you will grow new love by strengthening the food of love—attention. You'll ignite your relationship with freshness and appreciation. Look how you have already tended to your relationship in preparation for tonight: You've scheduled pleasure together, shared daily meditations, contributed items to your Sensual Space, prepared a clean mouth and body, and showed up on time. Tonight you will practice hearing, seeing, touching, sensing, and kissing your partner with sacred attention. Attention feels good, and deep attention is blissful.

Erotic Exercise 1: Opening Ritual   [FIFTEEN MINUTES]

Begin this journey ceremonially by lighting candles, playing sensual background music, and preparing your Sensual Space in silence as if you were an ancient temple priest or priestess. Enter the space wearing loose clothing, or none at all if you prefer. Sit facing one another with pillows propped up to support you comfortably.

Mark the beginning of the evening ritual with a Heart Salutation (a simple bow of appreciation with your hands in prayer position at your breastbone). Notice how your body responds to the power of childlike ritual that speaks to us on a level deeper than words. Now work with the following exercises.

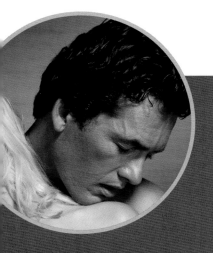

"Just the opening ritual with Ocean Breathing took me to a new place with my lover; **we melted together.**"

—REESE, AGE 43

CREATE SENSUAL SPACE TOGETHER

Together you will purify your space by cleansing it of qualities you wish to get rid of and sanctifying it with qualities that you choose to invite in. With the focus of spiritual shamans, set the timer for ten minutes and follow these three steps:

1. **Clear negative energy.** Take turns naming negative fears and doubts you have brought into the space and are willing to release. For example, say, "I let go of my worries from the day," or, "I rid myself of expectations for this evening," or, "I expel my fear that I will not be able to do the exercises well," or, "I expel my inhibitions and regrets from this space." Gesture with your hands the idea of "away" to wave each doubt out the room's door or window. Involving the body in this way speaks on a deep level. Keep taking turns naming and ridding the room of negative energies until you are both finished. The power of these negative energies begins to dissipate immediately.

2. **Call in positive energy.** Feel the space created in the room with negativity expelled. Now fill the newly created void with your positive affirmations. Take turns calling in qualities to enhance the room or container for your loving exploration. You may say, "I call in compassion," or, "I call in love," or, "I invite my playful child in," or, "I invoke my sense of discovery and curiosity." Use your body to motion in these luscious attributes to make your space sacred and safe; outstretch your arms and bring them to your body in a gathering-up gesture and pour it over your heads. When you call love into your room, you both are literally "in love."

3. **Speak your intention.** After the space is cleared of negative energy and charged with positive energy, share your personal intention for the evening. You may say, "I intend to experience from an open heart," or, "I intend to stand strong in uncertainty," or, "I intend to be aware of my breathing [or sensations]." Articulate one short, positive statement to guide your adventure.

COME INTO THE BODY WITH OCEAN BREATHING

After creating Sensual Space, eye gaze and Ocean Breathe together as practiced in the Daily Erotic Ritual, but extend it to five minutes. Set the timer. Add a Heart Hold: Place your right hands over each other's heart and your left hands over the hand that rests over your heart. With each breath, let your awareness sink deeper into your body, and drop your attention into your expanding and contracting chest. Ride the sound of your breath. Keep your belly soft. As you slow and deepen your breath, imagine sending energy from your heart through your arm and hand into your partner's heart. End with a Heart Salutation (a simple bow of appreciation with your hands in prayer position at your breast bone).

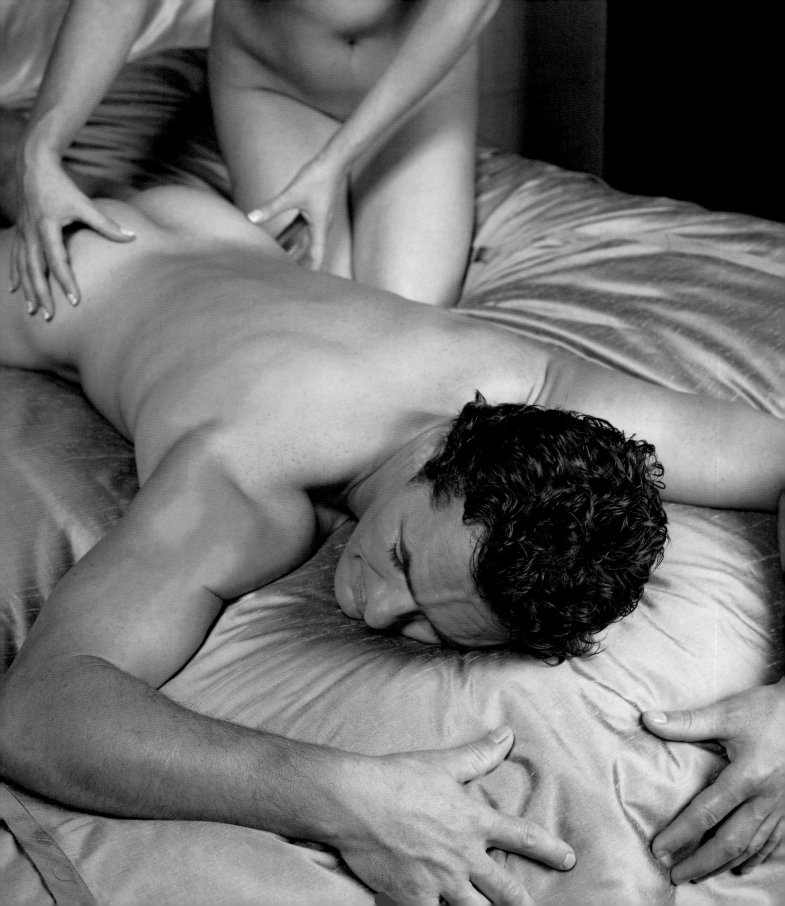

Erotic Exercise 2: Hearing Your Partner with Attention   [FIFTEEN MINUTES]

When I returned from living a full year in Mexico with a native family, my friends asked me whether I had become "fluent" in Spanish. We value being active (talking) up north, but farther south, where relationships are central, people value listening (passive). I suggested to my friends that a better question would be, "How well could you understand what others were saying after a year?" A baby listens long before it begins to speak. We all need to be heard; listening to your partner is a natural first step in intimacy.

LISTEN WORD FOR WORD

Sitting across from one another, decide who will be active, or the speaker, first. Pick some mundane subject to talk about, such as how to take out the garbage or how to put a worm on a hook, etc. The active partner will talk, clearly and deliberately, for ten seconds on this subject. When the timer sounds, the listening partner will feed back word for word what he or she has heard. Aim for precision. The active partner will probably let you know what you missed. Have fun. Then trade roles. After both of you have had a turn at exact listening, take a minute to share what the exercise was like for you. How was it to try to recount word for word? How was it to be listened to so exactly?

LISTEN FOR ESSENCE

Trade being the active person first and choose another neutral subject, like describing a favorite pet or vacation. This time, speak for thirty seconds, and ask the listener to reflect the essence of what you said back to you, not particularly the exact words. Set the timer

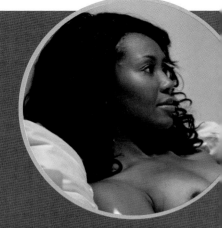

"**I felt so honored** to hear my partner reflect back to me what I said without any evaluation or judgment—just rephrasing what I said. I realize how giving and receiving attention is the backbone to great loving. **Attention melts me to my very core.**"

—RONDALYNN, AGE 39

and begin. At thirty seconds, wind down your last sentence. The listener now paraphrases the discourse in his or her own words, catching as many of your points as possible. Give the listener feedback as to accuracy or anything he or she may have missed. Trade speaker/listener roles.

After you both have had turns listening for essence, discuss for a few minutes what insights you gained from this exercise in deep listening. How does it feel to have someone closely reflect your words back to you? How well could you listen? How could you improve? How does deep listening feel to you in your body? How well do you usually listen to those around you and to your partner?

Erotic Exercise 3: **Seeing Your Partner with Attention** [TWENTY MINUTES]

All of us have walked into a room and felt attention turn to us. Maybe you've been at a party and, from across the room, someone's eyes met yours just for a moment, making you feel a "ting" or jolt in your body. How does it feel in your body to "get" attention? How does it feel to "need" or even try to "grab" someone's attention?

Look at each other with your longing-for-attention look, and exaggerate it. For fun, try to "grab" your partner's attention; be childish about it. Then try the opposite. We know how it feels to be lavished with attention; show the face of being totally lapped up with gushing attention. Attention registers deeply in our sensing body. In the next exercise, which I learned at a couples intimacy workshop with Richard and Antra Borofsky, you will take turns sending and receiving attention to enhance the depth of your attention.

- **Sending attention:** To send attention, you need to first be able to assess what you can truly give at any moment. Face it, sometimes you do not feel loving. Sometimes you don't have the energy or desire to give attention, and it's best to recognize it. Without judging yourself, tell your partner, "Right now I'm too [depleted, tired, distracted, etc.] to be able to give you attention." It's better to Come Clean than try to fake it.

- **Receiving attention:** Sometimes you are not able to receive attention, even though you want it desperately. If you are stressed and fretting, "Do you love me? Do you love me? Tell me you love me," someone could tell you, "I love you," and you'd still not accept it.

To receive attention, you need to open up a space in the body for the attention. You need to physically relax and soften the space around your heart to take it in. Opening the heart to receive your partner's attention happens by letting go of past disappointments, fears, and judgments you hold against him or her. It's no simple task; you must choose to let go of your need to be right and any resentments you hold toward your partner. Are you willing to receive a beloved in the moment, unencumbered by the past?

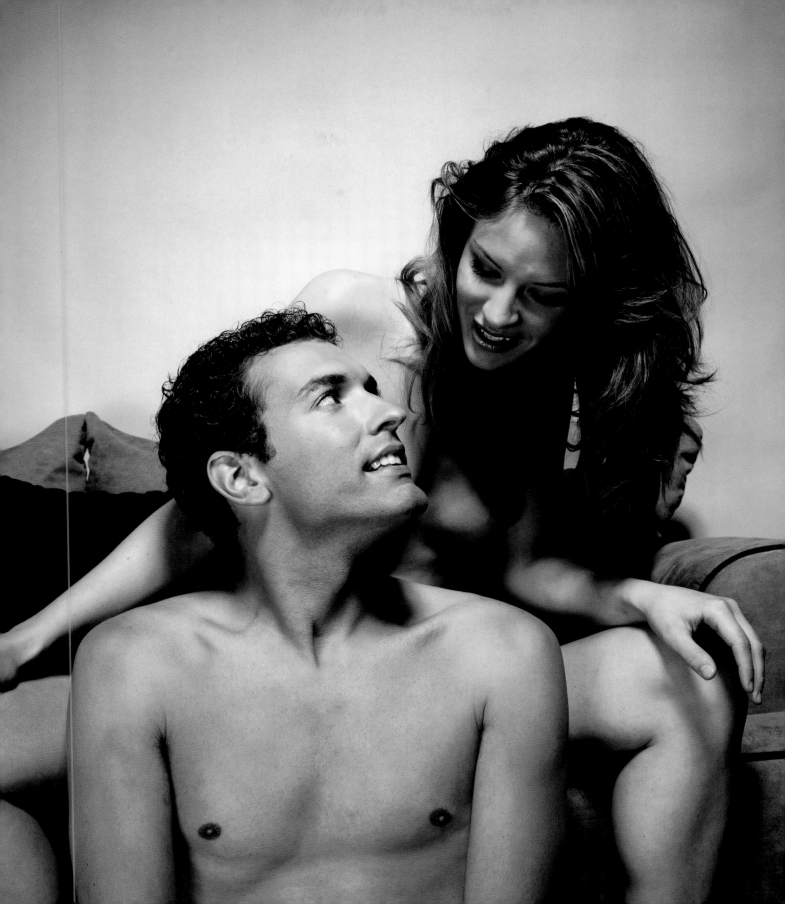

The most gracious and sweet gesture of any relationship is choosing to open your heart and receive the other with freshness and wonder of your childlike being. In choosing to consciously give and receive deep attention, you both become pilgrims seeking a new path, stepping onto unknown shores, and pioneering a new relationship world.

SEND AND RECEIVE

Sit facing one another with your hand over your partner's heart, like in Ocean Breathing. Assess whether you are able in this moment to send full attention to your partner and whether you are willing to open your heart, relinquish past disappointments, and receive your partner's attention. Be true to yourself. If there's something preventing you from full attention in this moment, give it voice, or take care of it. How to Come Clean with your partner is covered in Erotic Night Two. Because you have set this time aside to tend to one another tonight, you are both probably eager to start. Signal your willingness to proceed by nodding to each other.

Decide who will be the sender first. Sender, breathe in deeply. With the inhale, imagine gathering up your most precious commodity—your attention—and with the exhale, imagine sending it into the heart of your receiver. Inhaling is good for gathering; exhaling is good for sending. Take several breaths. When you feel ready (don't hang onto your gift), send your attention out, speaking aloud the words "for you" so your partner can hear your heartfelt intent.

Receiver, prepare yourself by breathing deeply into your heart, imagining it growing bigger and softer. Breathe into the protective armor around your heart, and visualize it softening and falling away with each breath. When you hear your partner say, "For you," take in the sound of his or her voice, the offering of his or her precious gift of attention. When you feel it enter your heart, receive it fully, and say out loud, "For me."

Repeat sending with an audible "for you" several times more and receiving with the reply "for me." Gaze into each other's eyes, the window of the soul. When you feel complete, take a few deep breaths together, and bow in a Heart Salutation. Without talking, exchange sender and receiver roles. Silence helps integrate an experience, whereas engaging in small talk distracts you from your feelings. When you stay in your body with your feelings instead of going to your head with chatter, you assimilate instead of avoid the experience at hand, even if it makes you uneasy.

TALK ABOUT THE EXPERIENCE

After you have both practiced sending and receiving attention, take turns talking uninterrupted for two minutes (time it!) about what the experience was like for you. You may choose to share what you noticed in your body when you said "for me" and "for you." How was it different to give or to receive attention? Was one role easier for you? Did anything

The Rules for Touching

Touching is a powerful and endearing way to give and receive deep attention. Your skin is your largest organ, and it becomes more sensitive as you age. Also, your ability to focus attention and thereby magnify bodily sensations strengthens with age. Learning to touch from a place of deep attention transforms ordinary time and reality into prolonged erotic trance states.

These few simple guideposts will leave routine, habitual, and repetitive touch in the dust and teach you that touch is spontaneous and full of interest, discovery, and presence. Here are the Rules for Touching:

- **Take turns touching.** Often you may both be so busy touching each other at the same time that neither of you takes the time to enjoy your own pleasure. When you learn to take turns, as giver and receiver, you can begin to feel the smallest hint of your arousal. You have more space to enjoy the uniqueness of each sensation.

- **Touch for your pleasure.** Touching for your own pleasure versus trying to turn on your partner allows you to feel genuine joy instead of performance anxiety. Engaging in your own discovery, following your curiosity, and relaxing into your own sensations will encourage your receiver to do the same. Touch becomes playful. Instead of trying to take care of the other person, you get to sense your own body. You both become free to feel instead of pressured to perform.

- **Focus on your sensations.** Focus your attention solely on the point of contact where your skin touches your partner's, and follow each sensation, whether you are the giver or receiver of touch. When your mind wanders from the place of touch (and it will), gently bring it back, over and over, to focus again on your sensations. Sensate focus keeps you in your body moment to moment and reduces mind chatter that worries about the future or frets about the past.

- **Touch for the journey.** Touch without trying to get someplace, like hard, wet, or to orgasm. Outcome-oriented sex isn't play; it's work and not much fun. Remember playing as a child? Games meandered into long summer evenings, and there were no endings. You were mesmerized by the journey. Touch freely for the joy of the moment, and your partner will receive it that way.

change for you as you repeated the same words over and over? How do you feel in your body right now? After one of you speaks, the other takes a minute to reflect back on the essence of what was said without making any additional comments. Check for accuracy— you are learning a new skill. Exchange speaking/listening and reflecting roles.

Erotic Exercise 4:
Caressing Your Partner [FORTY MINUTES]

Caressing is really more sensual than sexual. Sensual touch is about enjoying the pleasure of the sensations in the moment, whereas sexual touch is more goal-oriented. The sensual touch of Erotic Nights is about becoming enthralled with the journey and building a reservoir of desire versus touch that has a destination, such as intercourse.

Decide who will give a caress first (the man in this example). Before you caress your partner, assemble various feathers, furs, scent misters, silk scarves, and cornstarch (yes, from the kitchen). Caress is not massage. You will not be manipulating the underlying tissue; rather, you will be lightly teasing the nerve endings of the skin.

The receiver, or touchee, makes herself comfortable lying down on her back or stomach, whichever she prefers, on the bed with pillows propped however she likes. She may choose to leave her clothes on or take them off: Remember, exercising choice without judgment empowers sexuality. Now set the timer for 20 minutes, and consider turning up the music slightly. Caress is a nonverbal activity that helps us move out of the head and into the body.

Begin by laying one hand gently over the sacral or abdominal area and the other hand over her heart. Hold still. Breathe together, making the sound of the ocean. When your Ocean Breathing is synchronized, move your hands slowly and lightly over her skin. Put a tablespoon of cornstarch on your palms, and rub them together for the silkiest touch ever. Spread this angelic dust in long, continuous, smooth strokes from head to toes, letting your breath lead your movements.

Lighter and slower are better. Caressing is a case where less is more. On a touch scale of 1 to 10, soft to hard, feminine touch is 1 to 5 and masculine is 5 to 10. Stay in the range of feminine touch, which often is overlooked in a rush to the finish line in sex. Tease her

Taking turns giving and receiving allows each of you to feel more sensation.

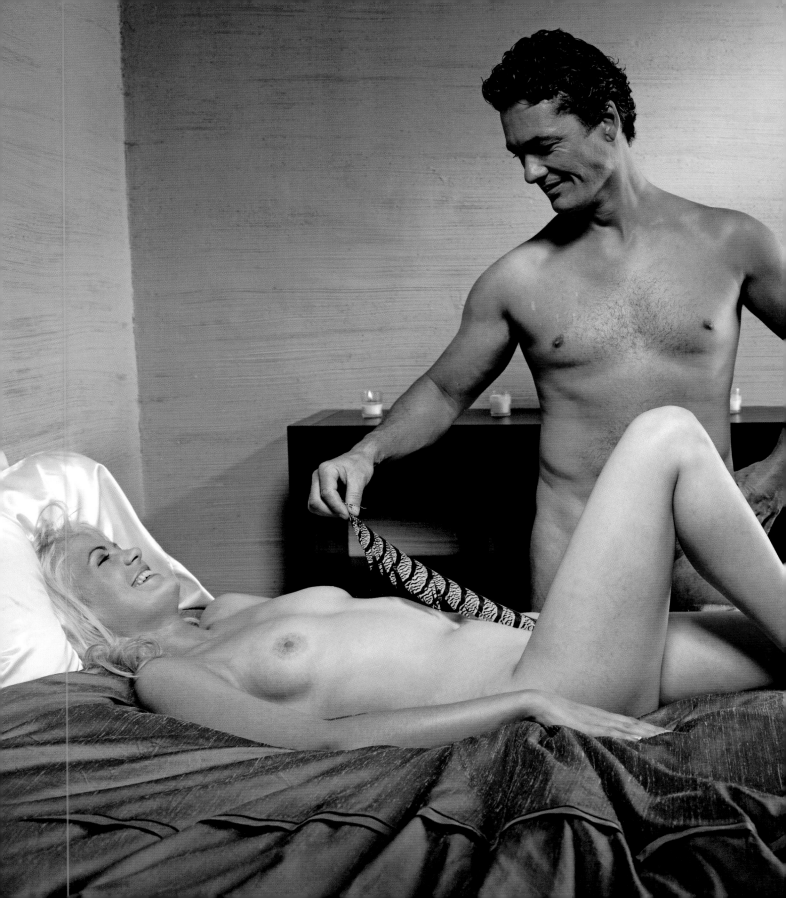

with a feather and fur. Pause. Breathe. Stillness is a stroke. Intimacy grows in the pauses, passion in the action. A musician knows that without the rests, there is no music.

Float a silk scarf over her body, or mist her from afar, and let the droplets drift over her skin. Brush over the genitals, but do not linger there; you are awakening the whole body as a large erogenous zone. Encourage desire by being a subtle and skillful orchestrator of sensual delights. You are the patient gardener, growing love and nudging the sprouts of fledgling desire toward the daylight.

Be mindful of the Rules for Touching (page 39) while touching for your wonder, focusing on your sensations, and meandering freely. Like any other practice, the more you do it, the more naturally your attention will rest on each sensation, and the joy will rejuvenate you both. When the timer sounds, marvel at how focused attention to sensations can suspend time.

Ecstasy by definition is simply "standing outside of stasis or the normal." Recognize your natural ability for moments of ecstasy. Take a few deep breaths together, share a Heart Salutation, and switch roles. You may also try adding occasional (timed) caresses during the week, and extend a Daily Erotic Ritual with a two-minute face, hand, or foot caress.

Adding Touch to Your Daily Erotic Ritual

On occasion and by mutual consent, you may extend the Daily Erotic Ritual by adding an exchange of sensual, nonsexual touches at the end of Ocean Breathing. Ask your partner, "Would you like to extend the Daily Erotic Ritual for some touching?" When responding, say "yes" only if you can truthfully extend your attention longer without other concerns pulling at you. Extending time works only when both partners agree. If your partner replies, "No, thank you," graciously return a "Thank you." A "no" has more to do with what's happening within your partner than to do with you or your technique.

If you mutually consent to exchanging caresses, ask, "Where would you like to be touched?" Hands, shoulders, neck, hair/head, and feet are good places for caresses. Set the timer for two minutes. While caressing, Ocean Breathe, and practice the Rules for Touching (page 39): Take turns, touch for your pleasure, focus on your sensations, and touch in the moment without goals. Exchange roles after two minutes. Exchange a Heart Salutation and come apart. If you wish a longer caress, certainly ask for it, but not in connection to the Daily Erotic Ritual. Keep the timeframe boundaries of the Ritual intact.

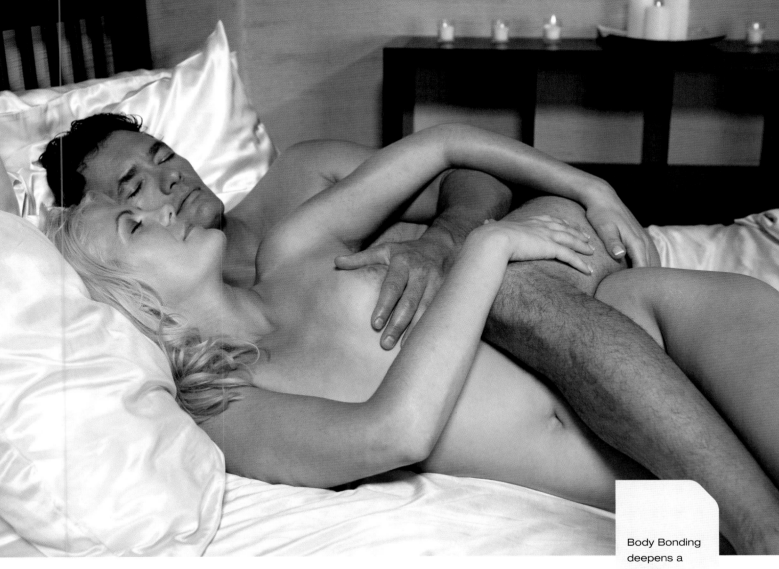

Erotic Exercise 5: Breathing and Attention:
Body Bonding [TWENTY MINUTES]

What looks like inactivity on the surface is perhaps the most profound of all focused erotic attention exercises. Body Bonding with your partner opens your energy channels at a subtle level where the boundaries between bodies begin to dissolve and merge. You learn to expand attention to bodily sensations as they metamorphose, moment to moment, and to notice the subtle building and dissipation of desire without needing to judge or act on it.

1. **Find a comfortable place to lie together,** such as on a bed; set the timer for twenty minutes; and play soft, relaxing music. You can lie together in a Spooning position (chest to partner's back), or the lighter partner can lie on top of the heavier one's back or front. Make sure you are comfortable and supported by pillows where needed.

Body Bonding deepens a formless, relaxed, and merged space with your partner.

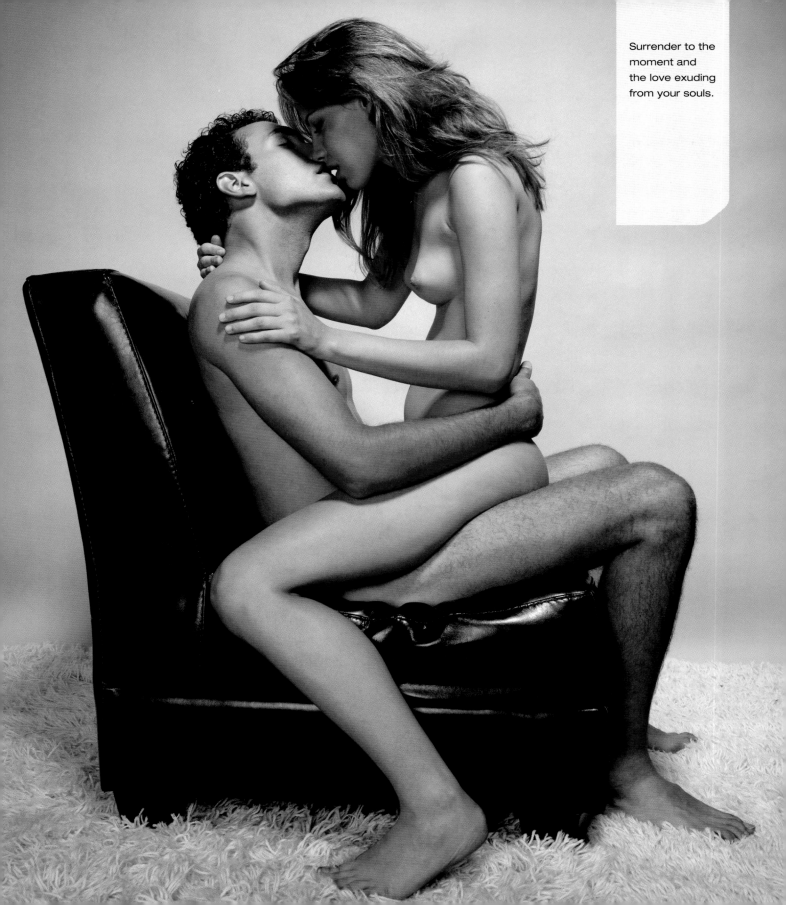

Surrender to the
moment and
the love exuding
from your souls.

2. **Once lying together, begin to be aware of your breath,** letting your worries and tension fall away with each exhale. Exhaling, imagine expelling your fears, resentments, and expectations. Release the need to think and analyze. Let your tongue float freely in your mouth, not touching the any part of the mouth cavity.

Observe your partner's breathing rhythm. Are you beginning to synchronize? Notice all the details of how your bodies feel together—the heat, the softness, the gentleness of being together, the feelings of protection and safety. With each breath, let yourself fall deeper into the body, becoming transparent and feeling the vulnerability of the present moment and the wonder of uncertainty. Feel this new reality where doing and not doing are one, and where giver and receiver are one.

Can you feel your boundaries dissolve into the other? Can your heart open and welcome the other in? Let the exploration be effortless. Can your spirits float away beyond the boundaries of the body? Usually it takes fifteen to twenty minutes (or longer) to deepen into this formless, relaxed, and merged space. Be patient. Even great sex needs to be practiced, so repeating this exercise is helpful.

A common mistake is to expect too much too soon. Enjoy the journey. Make sure you feel free to gently readjust your position while Body Bonding. Your partner won't feel disturbed by your movement but rather glad that you are making yourself comfortable. End with a Heart Salutation and mutual sharing of the experience. Body Bonding is a stepping stone to sexual bonding. It can be done in the same spirit while genitals are connected, which is something you may choose to do on another night.

Erotic Exercise 6: Experiencing the Tantric Kiss   [TWENTY MINUTES]

Breathing in and out with each other while kissing is a divine exchange of essences and an easy route into altered states of consciousness. Prepare by brushing your teeth or taking a breath mint.

1. **During this exercise, the woman sits on the man's lap,** head above his, in the classic Tantric yab-yum position, with her feet touching behind his body. The man should do the same if he is flexible enough. Set the timer for eight minutes.

2. **Gaze into your partner's left eye,** which is the tunnel into the soul, and bring attention to your breathing. Listen for your partner's breath, and ease into a joint rhythm.

3. **When your breathing is synchronized, loosely put your lips together** with open air spaces so suction is not formed. Breathe in and out together simultaneously through loosely connected mouths. Your eyes may be open or closed, or you may alternate between them. Feel how each breath goes in cool and comes out warm. Feel how each breath goes in dry and comes out moist.

Be willing, as in Body Bonding, to let yourself go into an erotic trance, that timeless place of surrender to the wonder of the present moment. When the mind wanders from the sensations of your mouth-to-mouth breathing, gently bring it back, over and over. Discipline the mind from chatter by simply bringing it back to your bodily sensations. Refrain from active moving in the kiss.

Alternate breathing: At the end of eight minutes, reset your timer for another eight minutes to begin the most intimate breathing yet. After a minute or so of resuming in-sync breathing in a soft, loose kiss, the man will change his breath to be opposite the woman's: When she's breathing out, he breathes in, etc. In this stage of the Tantric Kiss, your breathing is alternating and you are literally taking each other deeply inside yourselves. You are taking the sustenance of life from the other and returning it to your beloved with your love and blessings.

Allow yourself to feel the timelessness of this ritual and the ancient air exchanged between you. You are the temporary dancers in the continuous larger cosmic flow. Be humbled and appreciative of your brief embodiment. Be aware of all who have breathed this same air before you and those not yet here who will breathe it when you are gone. End with a Heart Salutation and sharing if you would like.

Erotic Exercise 7: Closing Ritual   [TEN MINUTES]

Design your own closing ritual to mark the movement from the sacred into ordinary reality. Be willing to come apart cleanly and without guilt. In becoming individuals again, you may feel selfish to separate after sharing so intimately. Yet without coming apart, you cannot come back together. Making up a simple ritual helps you make a clear and precise transition.

Decide, for example, on doing a gesture like three claps and a wink or reciting a favorite saying and stomping your feet three times. Designing a ritual is fun and childlike. After your short ritual, blow out the candles, and leave the space.

Remember to respect your vow to keep what happens in your Sensual Space only in that space. Remember your commitment not to have intercourse on Erotic Nights. You are building the foundation for truth and trust on this night, so honor it as a stepping stone. Let the experiences simmer, write in your Ecstasy Journal, or rest peacefully in each other's arms.

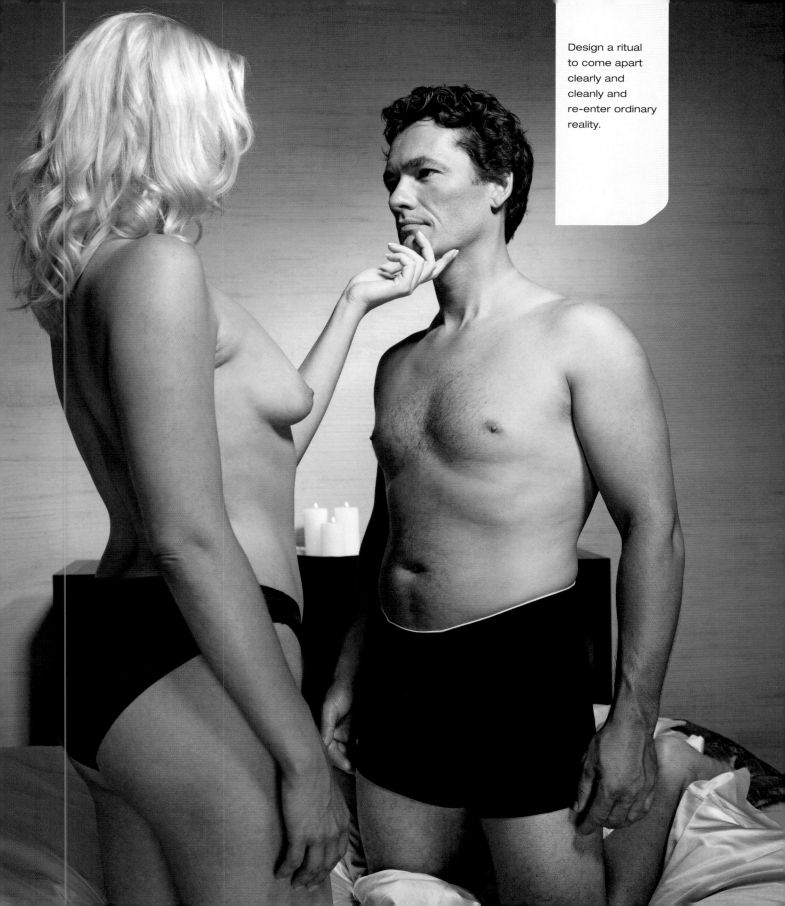

Design a ritual
to come apart
clearly and
cleanly and
re-enter ordinary
reality.

Looking Ahead

Sometime before the next Erotic Night, which focuses on truth telling, make two lists in your Ecstasy Journal of Things I Never Would Tell My Partner. Write a list of all the things you feel about him or her—things that you don't like but never would have the nerve to say. Remember this list is for you only, so include even the most detailed and difficult information. On another Journal page, make a list of things you never want your partner to know about you. Again, this list is for you. It should take about twenty minutes to write both lists.

Read Erotic Night Two several days before it takes place.

Erotic Recap

- Opening Ritual: *fifteen minutes*
- Hearing Your Partner with Attention: *fifteen minutes*
- Seeing Your Partner with Attention: *twenty minutes*
- Caressing Your Partner: *forty minutes*
- Breathing and Attention: Body Bonding: *twenty minutes*
- Experiencng the Tantric Kiss: *twenty minutes*
- Closing Ritual: *ten minutes*

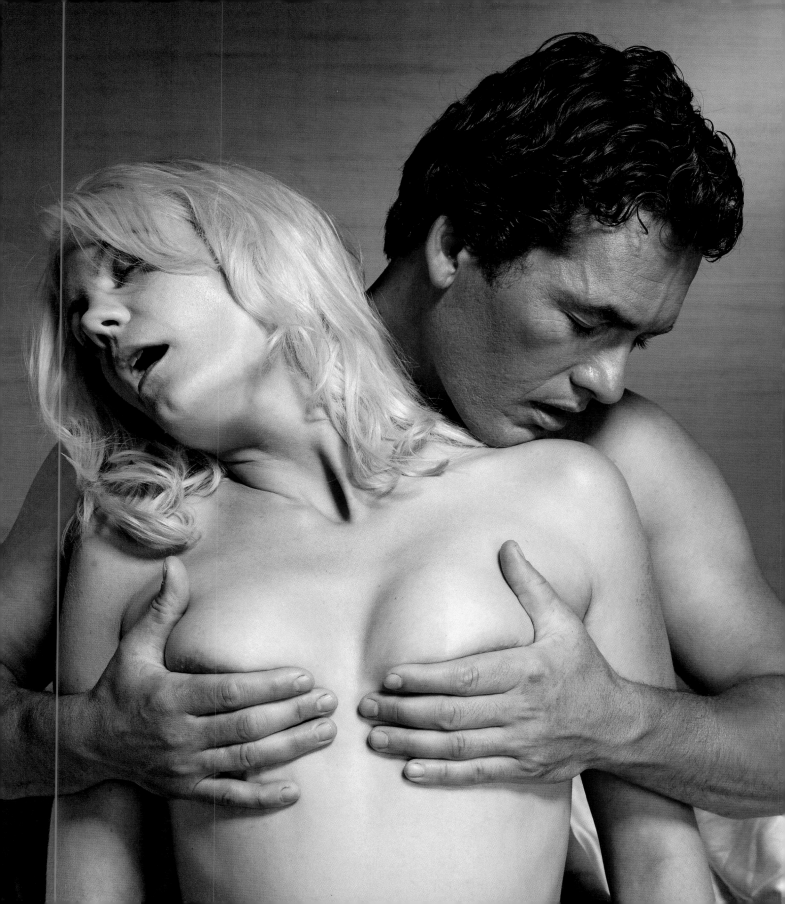

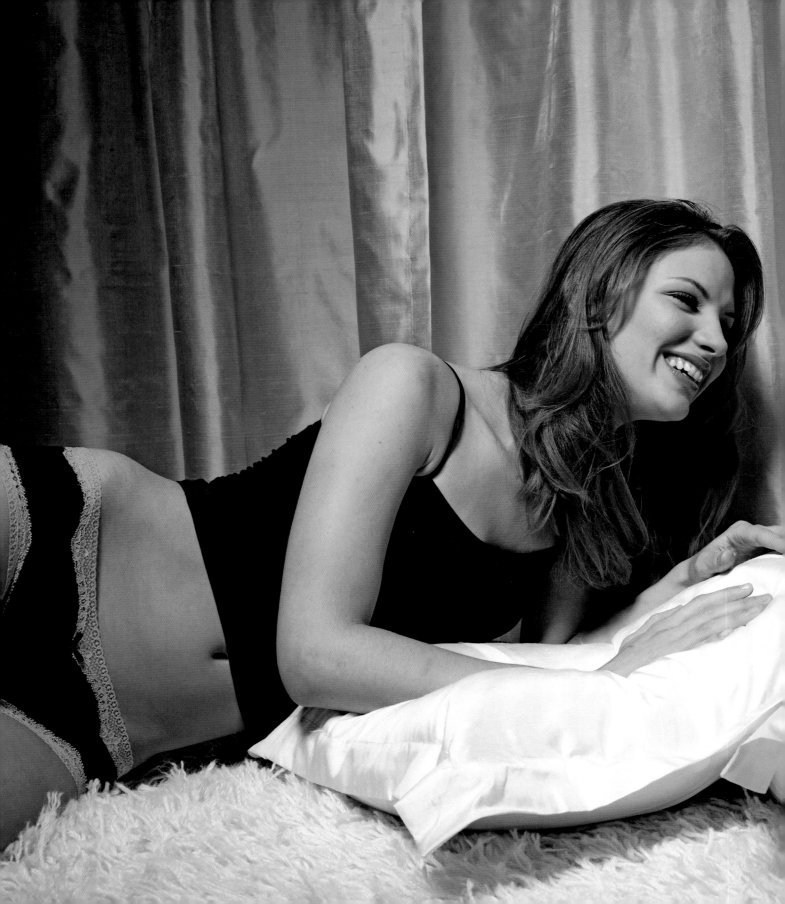

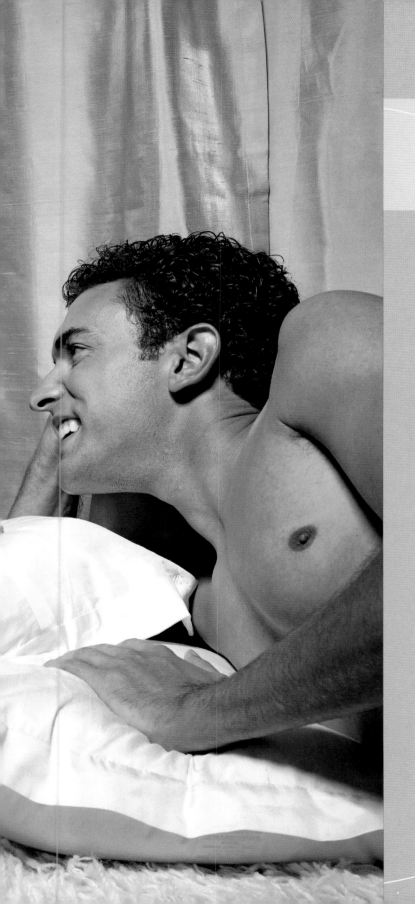

EROTIC NIGHT
TWO

Using
Honesty as
an Aphrodisiac

EROTIC NIGHT TWO

On your first Erotic Night, you learned to give and receive quality attention, the kind that makes you feel heard, seen, touched, sensed, and even kissed right down to your core. Tonight you will explore how truth is hot in the bedroom and the cornerstone for any juicy relationship. You will practice mutual honesty in clearing withholds, kissing, saying yes and no, and massaging your partner.

Prepare for your second Erotic Night by eating lightly, drinking lots of water, exercising, cleaning your body and mouth, dressing ceremonially, and showing up on time (review the "In Preparation: Readying Your Mind and Body" section on page 21). Each of you should bring your Ecstasy Journal complete with your two confidential Things I Never Would Tell My Partner lists, one list about her and the other about you (see "Looking Ahead" on page 48).

Erotic Exercise 1: Opening Ritual   [TWENTY MINUTES]

With your partner, prepare your sensual space with soft lighting, music, burning incense, candles, and so on.

1. **In a ceremonial manner, sit opposite each other and, if you have not already done so today, each give a two-minute Weather Report.**

2. **Continue to create your Sensual Space by clearing away negative fears, naming them one by one, and waving them out the door.** Proceed by calling in positive affirmations to sanctify the space, gesturing them in with your hands. Enjoy your inner child, who delights in ritual. Set intentions to give shape and direction to your evening, such as, "I intend to support myself in taking risks," or "I intend to be present with my partner," or "I intend to let go of judgment for the evening." Keep intentions short and positive.

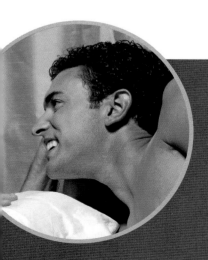

"I'd never really felt the details of Laura's hand like that before, even though I've held it for years. Each part felt so unique; **it was like feeling it for the first time.** To honor her in this simple and unrushed way was powerful and humbling."

—DANIEL, AGE 36

3. **Become conscious of your breathing,** slowing and deepening the breath. As you make the sound of the ocean with your breathing, gaze softly into your partner's left eye. Enjoy this familiar exercise (from your Daily Erotic Rituals) of coming into the body by inhaling together—bringing in with the breath all that you need, such as love and warmth, and exhaling together—letting go of all you don't need, such as tension and worry.

A Hand Caress allows you to cherish your partner in a wordless, soft space of appreciation.

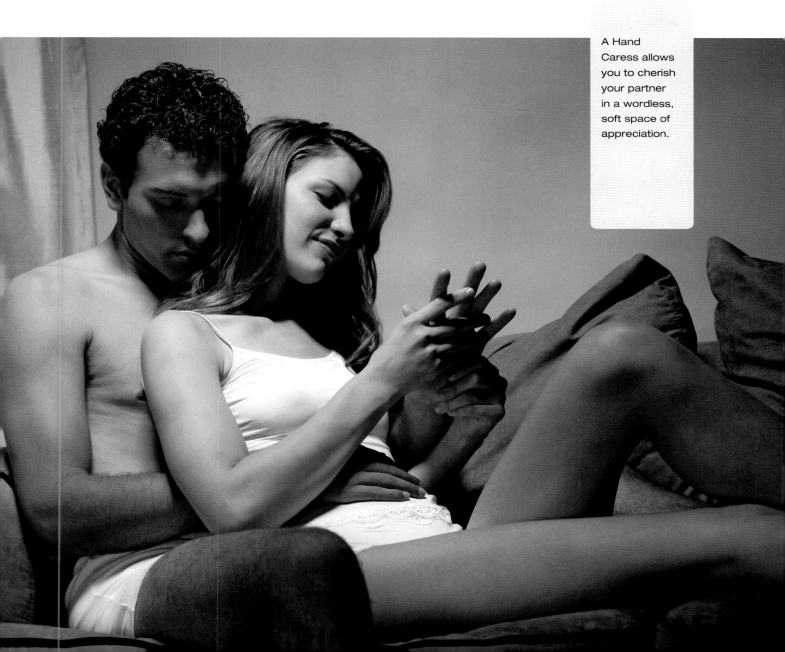

4. **After several minutes of slow, synchronized breathing, set the timer for five minutes, and take the hand of your partner into yours for a Hand Caress.** Close your eyes, and feel the heat and weight of this precious hand. Remembering the Rules for Touching (page 39), begin exploring the hand with your attention focused on your pleasure, feeling attentive to your sensations and free of any expectations.

5. **Slowly and lightly touch the outer contours of the palm and fingers, and move gradually to caress the entire hand, discovering every nook, mound, and fold.** Cherish this hand that works serving the community, supporting the family, and touching you lovingly. As the receiver, let your hand rest effortlessly like a rag doll in your giver's hands, and focus on your sensations with each deep breath.

6. **Allow the touch to carry you both into a wordless, soft space of appreciation.** Right behind your controlling mind and its resistance to letting go awaits the delicious experience of erotic trance. Momentarily relieve your mind of the need to think and evaluate, and instead fill your being with the wonder of observation and surrender. When the timer sounds, reset it for five minutes and change roles active/passive. End with a Heart Salutation.

Erotic Exercise 2: Coming Clean with Your Partner   [TWENTY MINUTES]

Coming Clean is a form of truth telling that clears away obstacles so you can be more erotically present with your partner. Holding back and hiding a feeling because it's difficult to talk about, or because you feel you need to protect someone, distracts you from being fully present, juicy, and creative in the moment. What is not said can hurt you.

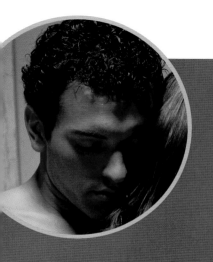

"I've discovered my own rule for Coming Clean with my partner. If something tugs at me uncomfortably, I take notice. If it comes back again, I say that's the second time. **If it distracts me a third time, I have to Come**

Coming Clean is saying difficult things in order to clear the air. It isn't about fixing anything or being right. It is about being honest with one another, taking risks, listening, and being with whatever emotions come up. If you and your partner practice Coming Clean often, you'll build a strong, fearless relationship.

Commit to this ritual routinely, and the truth will awaken and enrich your sex life. By adding Coming Clean to your Daily Erotic Ritual, you'll recharge your relationship daily. Honesty is an aphrodisiac; each time you release a withhold, each time you reveal your vulnerability, you enhance intimacy.

CLEAR THE AIR

Bravely announce, "I have a Come Clean." The response should be, "Go ahead" (if your partner has the time and attention to receive one). Speak in "I" statements for Come Cleans, and cover each of the following four steps, as outlined by Marshall Rosenburg in his book *Nonviolent Communication*:

1. **What you notice** (I noticed . . . facts surrounding the event)

2. **How you feel** (I felt . . . happy, sad, depressed, angry)

3. **What you need in this situation** (I need . . .)

4. **What you request of your partner** (I request that you . . .)

For example, partner one says, "I want to Come Clean about how I felt waking up in bed next to you this morning." Partner two says, "Go ahead." Partner one continues, "In bed I wanted to play around sexually. I quietly waited for you to initiate sexual play, and I noticed (1) you didn't make any sexual advances or moves toward me. I felt sad (2) because it seems to me I initiate play between us in the mornings most of the time.

Clean. Then I can return to the business of being fully present. Coming Clean has gotten easier for me, and I feel so good afterward. Surprisingly, **it brings clarity to my responsibility** in the situation."

—STEVE, AGE 42

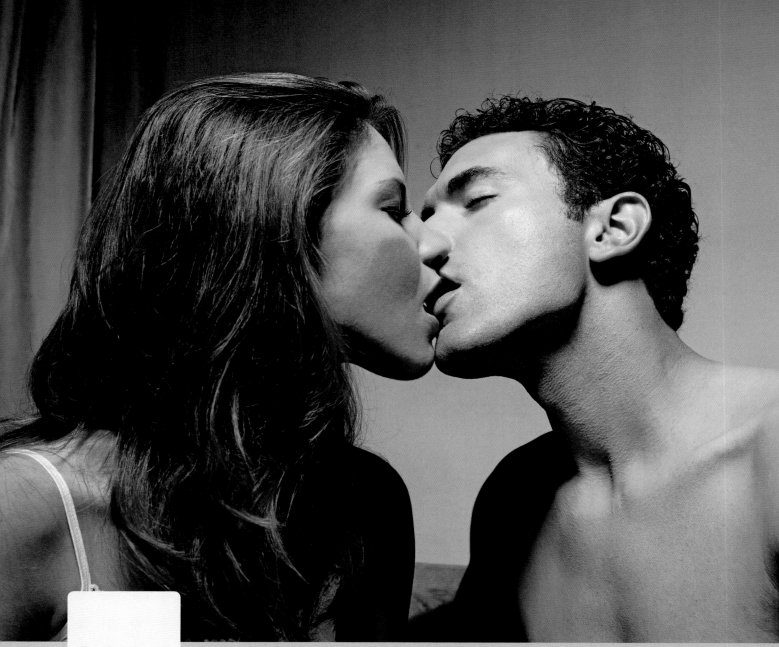

The kissing game teaches you to lead and follow in the game of love.

Taking the Lead

Taking turns gives each partner the chance to lead or design the show. Often the woman lets the man lead, because traditionally she sees her role as one of responding in sex. She may become bored with kissing and not know why. (Most likely, if one partner is bored, the other is, too.) She may not know that taking on the active role, or kisser, will spice up the show. Of course, the man needs to relax into the "kissee," or receiver, role. Most men love it when a woman takes charge, and there's nothing sexier than a woman taking her own pleasure.

I wondered why you don't initiate more. I need (3) to feel desired by you sexually, and I request (4) that you initiate sensual touching with me in the morning sometimes. I also wish you could read my mind and initiate sex with me just when I want it [smile]." Partner two responds, "Thank you."

Articulate all four steps, "I notice . . . I feel . . . I need . . . and I request. . ." with brevity and clarity. Stick to the facts, don't make assumptions, and avoid saying "you." The truth is short. State your Come Clean concisely, ideally within thirty seconds. Partners can help each other, especially at the beginning, with effective wording, which helps clarify the issue in each person's mind.

When receiving a Come Clean, simply acknowledge your partner's courage and commitment to the truth by responding, "Thank you." That is sufficient; being heard is powerful. No comment, no rebuttal, no blame, no defending oneself. It may trigger a future Come Clean from the you, but refrain from sharing it at this time. Later in the evening or the next morning, you may choose to Come Clean around the same or a similar issue. Keep tidy borders around the four-step format. Remember it's not about being right or fixing someone, it's about listening—powerfully.

Try sharing a Come Clean with your partner. Help each other if you are new to using "I" statements. For example saying, "This morning you didn't want to make love with me" is not a fact and doesn't use an "I" statement. Be "clean" about what you notice; this is a crucial part of the process. It's too easy to project or make up stories about the situation and believe them to be fact.

A Come Clean is more about the person coming clean than anyone else. Answer the question, "How does it feel in your body to give and receive a Come Clean?" You may want to commit to adding Coming Clean to the Weather Report portion of your daily meditation, or anytime you and your partner are willing.

Erotic Exercise 3: Playing the Kissing Game: Truth and Touch   [THIRTY MINUTES]

When you're true to what feels good to you, rather than being concerned with how it is received, you're telling the truth through touch. In the Kissing Game, you practice staying true to yourself while kissing your partner.

Kissing is another way to touch, so the same Rules for Touching (page 39) apply here. Instead of kissing each other at the same time, take turns being active and passive, or kisser and kissee. When you only have one thing to do, you are less distracted and feel more sensation.

1. **When you are the kisser, set the timer for ten minutes, kiss only the face and neck without touching the rest of the body, and find new ways to explore the sensations of your mouth and tongue for your pleasure.** When you are the kissee, make yourself comfortable, offer a slightly open mouth for the kisser's exploration, and do not react by moving. Close your eyes, and tune in to your sensations. Breathe.

2. **Start out slowly and leisurely with your kissing.** How lightly can you kiss? With a relaxed, soft mouth, graze over his or her cheeks, hair line, and facial features by barely touching the skin. Trace the eyebrows with soft lips or tongue. Tenderly kiss the tip of the nose, the corners of the lips, and the contour of the ear. The mouth is so sensitive that less is more. Your attitude should be inquisitive—play a new game with each kiss. Once you reach the mouth, kiss lightly without your tongue at first. Hard and wet mouth mauling misses the point. Discovery by tongue is a tender, playful journey.

3. **End with a Heart Salutation, then set the timer for two minutes, and have the kissee tell the kisser what he or she liked best about the kisses.** Use your Listening for Essence skills to become a better lover. Switch roles for another ten minutes of heaven. Again, take two minutes to tell your partner what you liked best about the kisses.

Erotic Exercise 4: Saying Yes and No Truthfully   [TWENTY MINUTES]

Saying yes to anything sexual when you feel obligated, want to pay back or manipulate someone, fear for your safety, are not sure what you want, or feel bored, is a detour on the road to great sex. To get back on your joyride, recommit to saying "yes" only for your enjoyment. "Maybe" is a no; only a clear "yes" is a go.

SAY YES WHEN YOU MEAN YES

Sometimes we don't say yes when we want something sensual or sexual. We're good at saying yes to other's needs but not our own. We're conditioned to think saying yes to our desires is selfish and bad. Self-denial becomes an art form. If asked, "Where would you like to go out for dinner?" Do you ever respond, "Where would *you* like to go?" In the bedroom, self-effacing is a recipe for disappointment.

Remember that a yes can become a no at anytime, anywhere, with anybody; you have the freedom to change your mind. If you don't feel this is a viable option with your partner, you're riding in the wrong car and headed in the wrong direction. You may think a shoulder rub is great one moment, but when a stroke becomes too repetitive or irritating (as inattentive touch can be!) you can decide to ask for something else. You may be well down a path to penetration sex and change your mind at any point. You have that right. And vice versa, a no can become a yes just as quickly. You're in charge.

SAY NO WHEN YOU MEAN NO

A functioning "no" in your sexual vocabulary is crucial for navigating the bumps, curves, and potholes along the road to great sex. "No" is a complete sentence. It needs no explanation, apology, or conditions. Receive your partner's no as a gift; respect it by responding, "Thank you." Dispense with defending your actions, offering regrets, or feeling resentment. Look at it this way: If your partner can't tell you no, what good is her yes? If you can't say no, your string of yeses is worthless dribble.

Think back to the last time a friend replied no to a request of yours. After your initial surprise (given our propensity to be pleasers), you probably felt put off. If the person held firm to her no and at the same time confirmed her respect and appreciation for you, then rejection may have turned into another emotion—lightness: "Gee, that was honest."

And then you become intrigued and interested—Wow, this person is real with me, there is value here, this relationship has possibilities. What, you may wonder, out of the hundreds of possibilities around this situation, could we both say yes to? A partner's no is the launching pad for mutual discovery—a platform to stage authentic play, a bowl in which to stir up a collaborate stew. We can decide to keep talking until we find what we do want to do together.

We often say yes to a partner when we mean no. We are afraid to lose our partner's love, lose the feeling of closeness, and perhaps lose the relationship. Fearing loss, we decide to not listen to our own truth and to instead do what our partner desires,

Women Especially Say No

Women are conditioned to say no to their desire for sex for many reasons. Sex is serious business for women. Besides ruining a reputation and spending the next twenty years raising a child (perhaps alone)—all from one little "yes"—marriageable women are conditioned to appear properly reluctant, shy, and innocent. Women grow up with the fairy tale that a man is going to rescue them and give them orgasms. He's got magic powers to read her mind (while riding a horse, of course!) and—if he loves her—presto! He'll save her from herself, or she can feed him to the dragons! Men are supposed to know, and women are supposed to shut up. Ladies (and Gentlemen), throw out the old tales, claim you desires, and always say yes to taking care of your sexual health and safety.

thinking this one time won't hurt. Then the one time becomes many, and we develop a habit of denying our own voice, especially when it comes to sex, where frequently shame silently runs the show.

Graciously Responding to a No

Hearing no from your partner is more about him or her than anything about you. Respond to her no with a gracious "Thank you." No is a jewel in the flower of an authentic relationship. It's an opportunity to keep talking until you get to a mutual, delicious yes.

SAY NO AND PRESERVE CONNECTION EXERCISE

Most of us need practice expressing a firm no while still offering approval and appreciation to our partner. In this exercise, you learn ways to preserve closeness in your relationship and still say no.

Start with one partner asking the other for permission to touch a body part, such as, "May I run my fingers through your hair?" Or, "May I kiss your vulva?" The receiving partner replies "No, thank you," and follows with a connecting phrase that acknowledges the courage and vulnerability of the requester. You can be firm in your boundaries and at the same time demonstrate that you value a close, continued connection. The following are examples of connecting phrases:

- "No, thank you. I think you are courageous to express your desire. I admire that about you."

- "No, thank you. I'm touched by your desire for closeness. I want to stay connected with your somehow."

- "No, thank you. I'm aware of your desire for connection, which I share. May I breathe and gaze into your eyes with you?"

- "No, thank you. I'm warmed by your desire for touch and connection with me. May I rest my hands in yours?"

- "No, thank you. Let's have some touching time later tonight after the kids are in bed; now is not a good time." (Refer to later only if you mean it; never lie just to put off someone.)

Take turns making five requests for touch, with the responding partner saying no followed by a connecting phrase. In requesting, be authentic; wait until you feel a desire to touch your partner and then ask to do it. In responding, choose from connecting phrases above, or make up your own. Make sure your phrase validates your partner's vulnerability and courage for asking. You may even envision a ray of light going from your heart into your partner's heart while speaking.

Counter offer another kind of touch in a connecting phrase only if it is authentically wanted by you. No mercy paybacks. Practice a couple of connecting phrases that do not offer touch. After each partner has said five no's with connecting phrases, discuss briefly what this exercise brought up for you.

How did it feel to be refused? Where in your body did you feel it? Could you stay in a caring space with your partner while refusing? Could you stay in a caring space when being refused? Did the connecting phrase help? Can you somehow convey to your partner, "You're okay, the touch you asked for is not"?

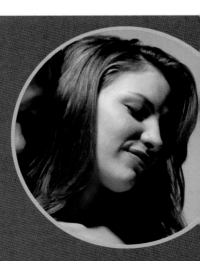

"Talking while touching really broke the ice for us. I found out great things about my partner, and **I loved being asked what pleased me, too.** I realized we never talk this way during intercourse. I see it as more possible now."

—ANNA, AGE 52

Erotic Exercise 5: Giving Foot Massages with Verbal Guidance [FIFTY MINUTES]

Touching is a gateway into the heart; however, if touch is routine, habitual, or unconscious, it can be distracting and even irritating. Touch is not about tolerating or enduring someone on our body. Touch is for enjoyment and ideally gets reinvented moment by moment. And just because we want firm touch one time doesn't mean we want it the next time.

FOOT MASSAGE EXERCISE

You may wish your partner could read your mind when it comes to being touched, and you've probably done a lot of guessing in giving touch yourself. During this massage, you will ask your partner for guidance in your touch, and he or she will express verbally what he or she likes.

Some may think asking how to touch someone feels too clinical, but desiring to serve a lover according to his or her wishes is a deeply caring gesture. Occasional verbal massages make future, nonverbal massages more exquisite. Decide who will receive first, and have the receiver settle comfortably in a reclined position with pillows under the knees. The giver gets the massage oil or lotion and sets the timer for twenty minutes.

Remember the Rules for Touching (page 39): Touch for your pleasure, focus on your sensations, and let go of goals to get somewhere. Pick up the first foot as you would a precious gem, and reverently cover it with oil. Unlike caressing, massage manipulates more than the nerves in the skin and goes deeper into the underlying tissues. After some stroking, check in with your partner, "Would you like more pressure or less pressure?" Respond to her answer simply with "Thank you." Ask again after adjusting your stroke. Keep checking in with your receiver during the massage with questions such as the following:

- "Would you like me to stroke faster or slower?"

- "Do you prefer longer or shorter strokes here?"

The Feet as Foreplay

The feet, rarely touched yet so sensitive, have receptors that are connected to our sexual organs. In essence, a good foot massage is foreplay, indirectly massaging the genitals. The feet become our "under-standing"; if you can stand up for what you want there, you can ask for what you want other places on the body.

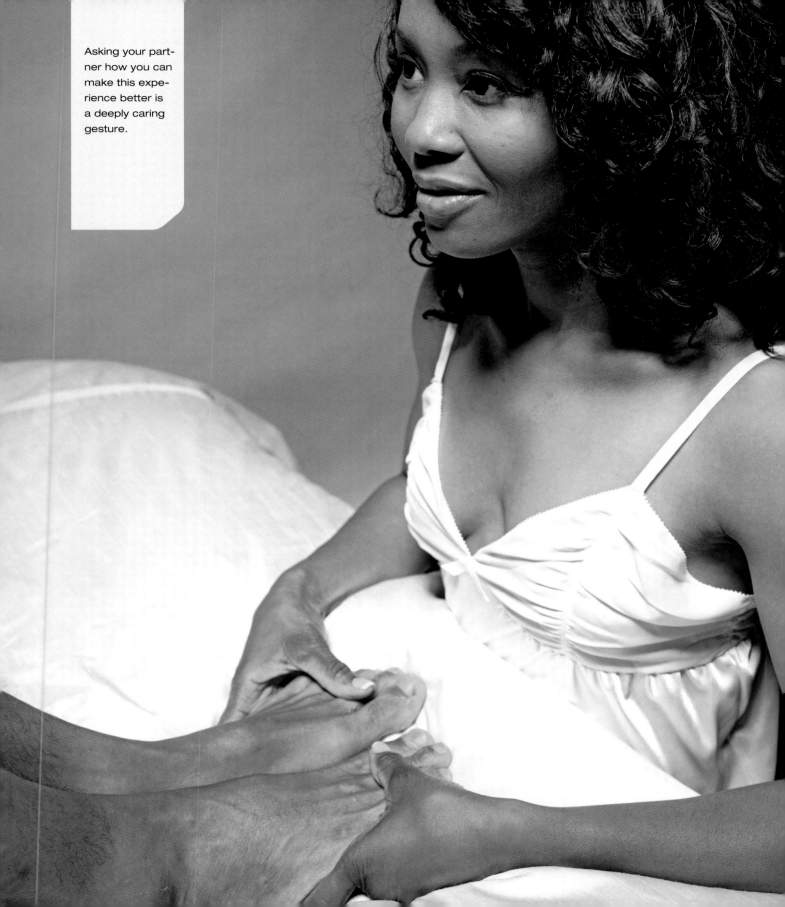

Asking your partner how you can make this experience better is a deeply caring gesture.

- "Do you want touch that's lighter or with more pressure?

- "What part did I miss or needs more attention?"

- "Do you like your toes pulled harder or softer?"

- "How could I make this experience better for you?"

Notice these are not yes/no questions. "Do you like this?" will likely pressure your part- ner to say yes when really you want instruction to help guide your touch. Halfway through, after about ten minutes, start massaging the other foot, and continue your verbal inquiry. Receiver, focus on your pleasure; take care of yourself, not the giver; and in addition to responding to your giver's questions, offer spontaneous feedback, such as, "Oh, I like that; try it softer," or, "Move more to the outside or top," or, "Please use . . . [more oil, less pres- sure, slower touch, etc.]," or, "Please change your stroke now." Appreciate your giver by saying, "That's yummy," or sigh with relaxation and happiness. At the end, take five minutes describe to your giver several "best moments" of the massage for you, and finish in a Heart Salutation. Trade roles, and reset the timer for twenty minutes.

Erotic Exercise 6: **Playing the Hot Seat Game**   [TWENTY MINUTES]

In this game, you get to ask all the questions you've never dared to ask before. It's fun to play, whether you've just met someone or have been with your partner for a long time. In life, when we answer a question, we can choose to lie, tell the truth, or not to answer. In the Hot Seat Game, your options are the same. Each of you gets to choose, in the moment, whether or not to tell the truth. Truth is a choice.

Don't Get Caught in a Habit

Look how habits work in our lives. Fold your hands together interlocking the fingers of your right and left hand. Which thumb is on top, right or left? Chances are you do it this same way every time, and if you were to try the opposite hand on top, it would feel awkward. Try it. Are you a creature of habit in your sex life too?

1. **Decide who wants to be on the Hot Seat first, set the timer for five minutes, and allow the person not in the Hot Seat to begin asking questions.**

2. **Ask your heart's desire—your wildest, funniest, sexiest, and most serious questions ever:** "What attracts you to me?" "What reservations do you have about our relationship?" "If you could spend a day and night being the opposite sex, what would you do?" "Where and when do you usually masturbate?" "Do you ever fake orgasms?" "What about sex frightens you most?" Unleash your curiosity and ask fearlessly. Remember that the questioner does not respond to any Hot Seat answers. He or she only listens.

3. **If the person on the Hot Seat is vague, you may ask for a specific example or a juicy detail.** When your question is answered, interrupt (if necessary) with "Thank you," and ask your next question. Maximize your time, don't let the speaker go on after you are finished listening; let your curiosity run the show. Most of us would choose to be empathetically interrupted by a listener than continue going on after he or she has the answer they were looking for.

Let your curiosity lead the show, unabashed and unashamed. At the end of five minutes, thank the person on the Hot Seat, bow in a Heart Salutation, and then reset the timer and trade roles! After you're warmed up, try a second round back and forth for another ten minutes. Remember to distinctly separate the active-talker and passive-listener roles.

Erotic Exercise 7: Closing Ritual   [TEN MINUTES]

Remember the Things I Never Would Tell My Partner lists you made in your Ecstasy Journals of things about him you can't tell him and things you can't tell him about yourself? Time performs magic on this list. You may want to Come Clean on something from this list now or in the days to come. If it feels is too risky, that's fine. Support yourself in your decisions. Just making the list was an act in truthfulness.

Looking Ahead

To prepare for the next Erotic Night, which addresses asking for what you want sexually, write in your Erotic Journal (at least a two nights ahead of time) on the topic of What Turns Me On Romantically. Write for ten minutes without putting down the pen (that's called automatic writing). Research your desires: What would you love to do with a partner? Where would you love to go? What would you love to give and receive from a partner? How do you like to be romanced? Write without thinking, write for yourself only, and write as if money and time were no issue. Have fun.

The second assignment is to write automatically for ten minutes on the topic of What Turns Me On Sexually. Picture an ideal encounter, and describe every last detail: where you are, details about your mate, the early sprouts of desire, growing arousal and stimulation, the juicy details of lovemaking, etc. Write to explore your desires, and keep your pen moving the whole ten minutes. Journal entries are for you only; sharing is a personal choice and never required.

Add Coming Clean to the Weather Report section of the Daily Erotic Ritual. Try playing the Hot Seat Game while dining out and waiting for your food to arrive. Warning: Others in the restaurant may jealously eye you and want a taste of what it is that you are doing!

Read Erotic Night Three several days before it takes place.

Design a closing ritual lasting only a few seconds, or use the same one from your first Erotic Night. Blow out the candles, and leave the Sensual Space remembering your commitments to confidentiality and the containment of sexual energy (nonpenetrating sex) for this night.

Erotic Recap

- Opening Ritual: *twenty minutes*

- Coming Clean with Your Partner: *twenty minutes*

- Playing the Kissing Game: Truth and Touch: *thirty minutes*

- Saying Yes and No Truthfully: *twenty minutes*

- Giving Foot Massages with Verbal Guidance: *fifty minutes*

- Playing the Hot Seat Game: *twenty minutes*

- Closing Ritual: *ten minutes*

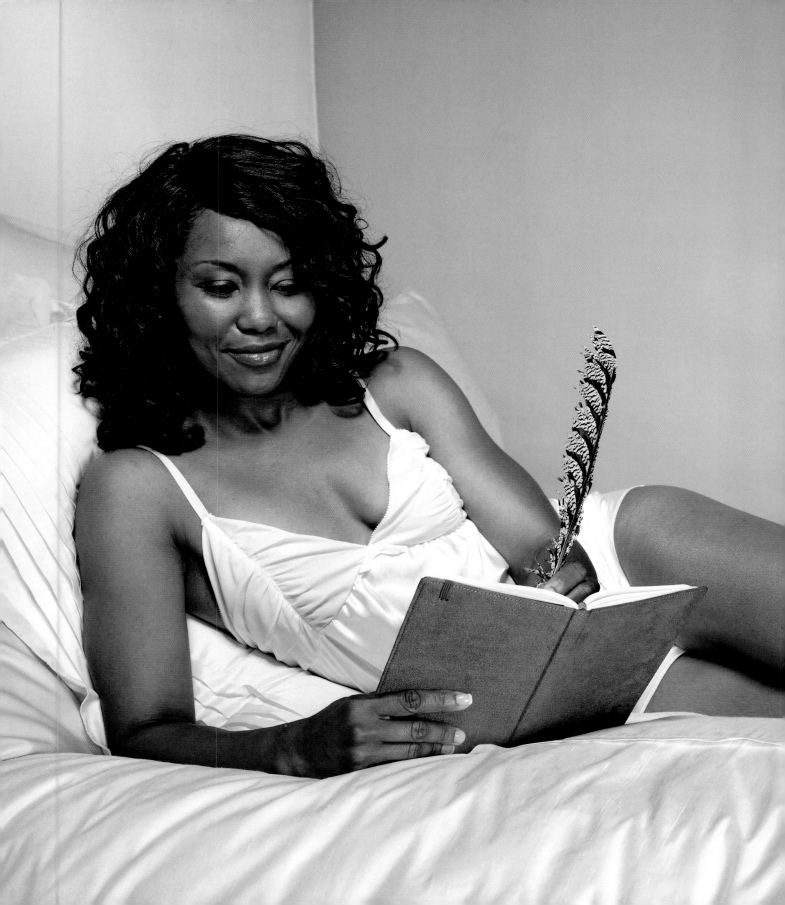

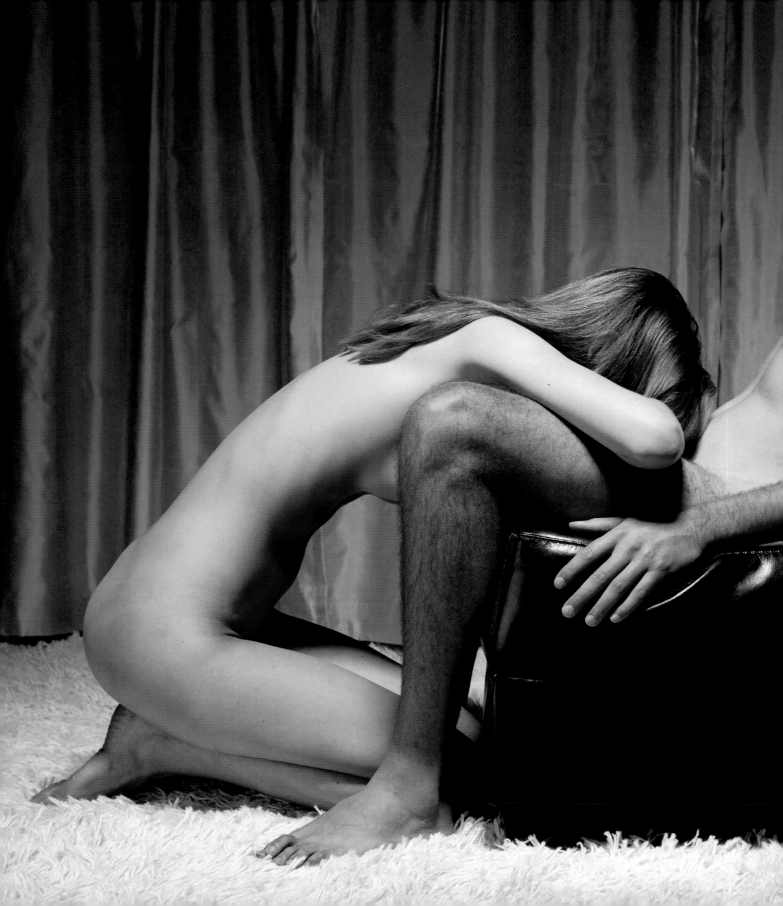

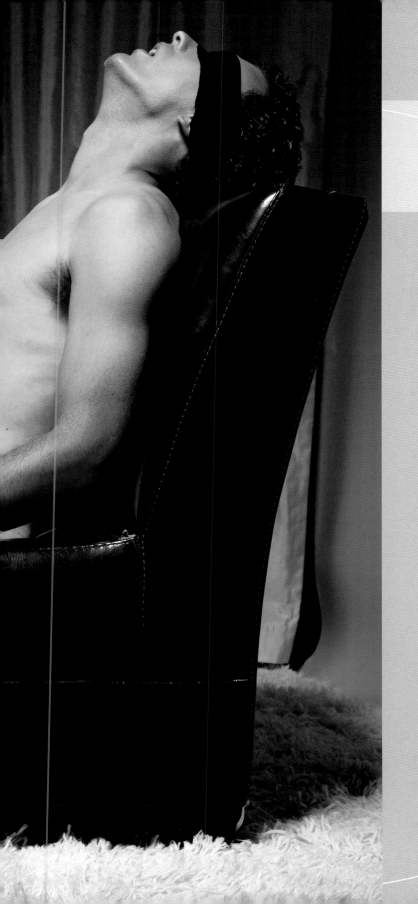

EROTIC NIGHT
THREE

Asking for
What You Want
100 Percent
of the Time

During the previous Erotic Night, you practiced telling the truth by Coming Clean, saying no to your partner with respect and connection, verbally guiding your partner during a foot massage, and playing the Hot Seat Game. Key to any rapturous relationship is being able to ask for what you want from your partner 100 percent of the time. Tonight you will explore expressing your desires.

It is easy to ask for what you want when ordering off the menu at a restaurant, or when asking a salesperson for something in a store. No shame there. But when it comes to sex, we find ourselves surprisingly silent about our needs. There are deep-seated reasons for this:

- **We deny our desires.** It's easier to cap our imaginations, pinch out the buds of our desires, and squeeze them to fit what we think someone else may want. We may censor our desires, thinking, "What would my partner think of me if he knew what I want to do?" We reign in our heart's desires, chastise ourselves for being wild and extravagant, and saddle ourselves to the mundane—the "right" way, the culturally "approved" way, and the already-tested way to act in our relationships. Before telling someone a heartfelt longing, we run a mental check on it: "How would my partner react? Is my desire something he would be willing to give me?" Our desires become removed from the source—ourselves—and evaluated instead on how they'll be received by others. Instead of taking care of you, you are trying to take care of your partner. Now is the time to learn to express desires without being attached to any particular outcome.

- **Desires make us vulnerable.** You probably find yourself holding back from expressing a need because you fear you'll seem needy, wanton, or weird. Desires make us vulnerable and transparent. Telling someone what you want means he or she may use it against you, ridicule you, and deny you of what you most want. Exposing desires can feel like

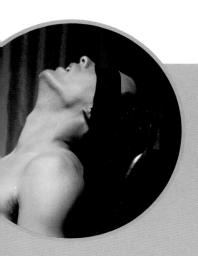

Tantra and Desires

Tantra, the ancient, Eastern art of sacred loving, offers a positive view of sexuality that celebrates sex and spirit, or body and mind, as complementary and integral components to enlightenment and fulfillment. Through our bodily senses and orgasmic joy, we fully realize our humanity, divinity, and connection with all creation. In Tantra, desires are synonymous with wholeness, health, and transcendence; desires are holy, and the sacred marriage of sex and spirit guides us into blissful union with ourselves, our lovers, and ultimately all life.

inviting some to walk over your soul in heavy boots. Expressing what you want feels like giving up power. It's easy to forget that being vulnerable can also enhance closeness with your partner.

- **We are shamed by our desires.** Being desirous is shamed in our culture, and most of us were probably taught that sexual wanting is selfish, a waste of time, addictive, immoral, unproductive, and dangerous. We grew up at war with our desires. Many religions view the body as a "distraction" from seeking spiritual truths; desires are base, and the pursuit of pleasure diverts one from the higher intellectual pursuit of God. The body is suspect, denigrated as inferior to the mind and spirit. No wonder we are embarrassed about having desires and have learned to keep them to ourselves. Instead, we need to welcome desires as a path to the divine and choose the Tantric positive view of sexuality. Instead of beating ourselves up over our desires, we can learn to welcome them. Commit here and now to freely expressing your desires without shame or fear. Stop judging your desires, or your partner's, and embrace them as guides to compassionate, erotic, spiritual growth.

Expressing desires doesn't mean you get what you ask for. Life is about (1) showing up, (2) paying attention, (3) telling the truth, and (4) being open to the outcome. Express your desires, and stay open to whatever happens. Put out your wishes without attachment to their fulfillment. Do not judge your partner's desires or his responses to your desires. Live honestly, and flow with what comes your way. Life is uncertain; stay open to the outcome.

Express your desires 100 percent of the time, and you will enliven your body, create spontaneity and zest in your relationship, and live passionately regardless of how others respond.

Erotic Exercise 1: **Opening Ritual**   [THIRTY MINUTES]

Having read about this night in advance, show up on time with a clean body and mouth, leave your knowledge at the door, and enter your Sensual Space with an open heart and a willingness to be present. Bring your Ecstasy Journal, which contains your two writing assignments, What Turns Me On Romantically and What Turns Me On Sexually (see page 65). With your partner, prepare your space with candles, music, etc.

1. **Sit opposite one another** and begin the evening's ritual with a ceremonial Heart Salutation followed by a two-minute (timed) Weather Report. At the end of the Weather Report, add a Come Clean, especially if you have not done so regularly in your Daily Erotic Ritual. Review the Coming Clean Exercise from Erotic Night Two (page 54) and use the "I notice . . . I feel . . . I need . . . I request . . ." format. Be concise and say "Thank you" after your partner Comes Clean without additional comments.

2. **Create Sensual Space** by releasing negative energy. Rid the space of all that may obstruct or detract from your erotic exploration, with statements such as, "I release my work-day hassles and worries."

3. **Set a positive intention** for the evening, such as "I intend to breathe deeply and enjoy being in my body." State your intention in one sentence with positive language; help your partner with wording if he or she uses the negative or gets too wordy.

4. **Come into the body** by setting the timer for five minutes and gazing into your partner's left eye. Breathe slowly and deeply, making the sound of the ocean with each inhale and exhale. You may choose to hold hands or put your hands over your partner's heart.

EXCHANGE A FACE CARESS

Touching the face is an endearing gesture of gratitude when done with attention and an open heart. Have your partner lie down with his head in your lap, using pillows for support wherever desired, especially under the knees. Set the timer for seven minutes, and close your eyes.

Cover his whole face gently with both of your hands, breathing with him and feeling the warmth. Slowly and lightly begin caressing his face by exploring with your fingertips his forehead and hairline. If his breath is shallow, breathe in his ear to remind him to let go deeper with each exhale.

Access your playful child in tracing the forehead, eyebrows, eyelashes, and contour of the ears. Leisurely follow the jaw line, and feel where the rough whiskers give way to the soft cheek. Touch lightly the lips, which naturally part like a baby's upon stimulation. Explore this unique face as if it were a treasure chest of riches; go where your fingers lead.

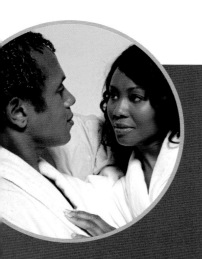

"At first I thought seven minutes was going to be a long time touching just the face of my beloved. **Then I got lost in its beauty.** For every joy, sorrow, and unknown we had experienced

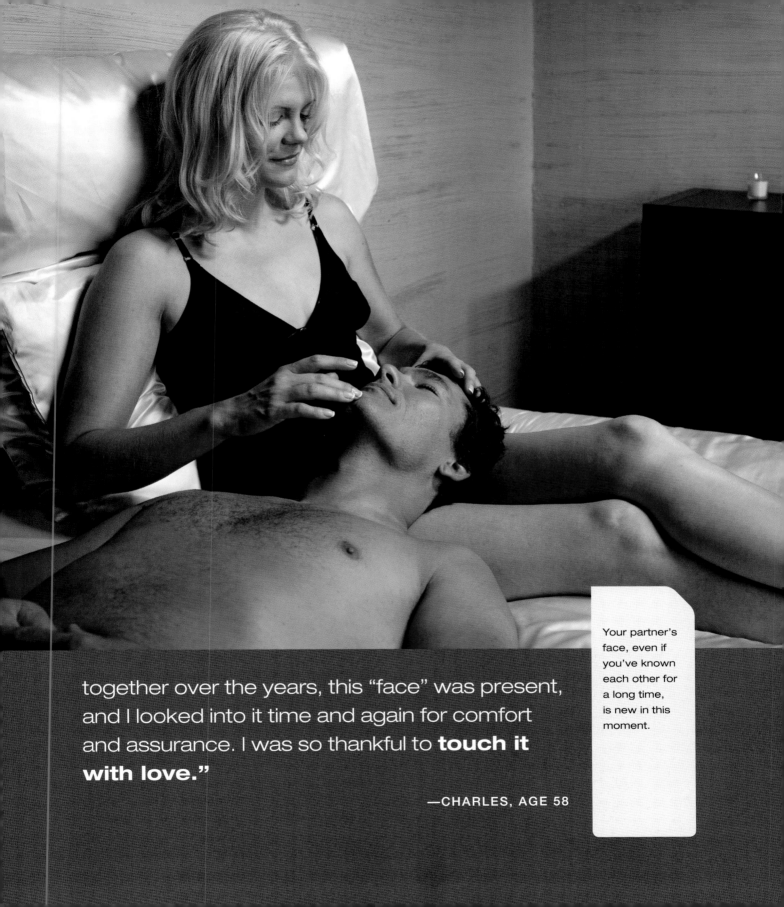

together over the years, this "face" was present, and I looked into it time and again for comfort and assurance. I was so thankful to **touch it with love."**

—CHARLES, AGE 58

Your partner's face, even if you've known each other for a long time, is new in this moment.

Lose yourself in the wonder of "seeing" him for the first time. This face, even if you've known each other a long time, is new in this moment. See aspects of the divine reflected in this face. Allow yourself to fall into an erotic trance and meander in this suspended, timeless realm. Slower is better; lighter is better. After the caress, ask him to tell you the best thing about the experience. Reset the timer and exchange roles for another seven minutes of erotic trance. End with a Heart Salutation.

Erotic Exercise 2: Playing the Three-Minute Game: Asking for What You Want   [FIFTEEN MINUTES]

The Three-Minute Game is a fun way to practice asking for what you want and getting permission from your partner before touching. You may not usually express desires out loud, yet it is very erotic. Hearing yourself speak what is generally silent gives validity to your fledgling desires. And being asked for permission to be touched by a lover may seem old-fashioned, but it's very hot.

ROUND 1: YOU ASK TO TOUCH YOUR PARTNER'S BODY (THREE MINUTES)
Choose who will be Yin (passive) and Yang (active) first. The Yang partner, in this case the man, sets the timer for three minutes and sits opposite his partner, connecting with her through breathing and eye gazing. Let your eyes gently wander over her body. Quietly notice when a desire to touch her nudges your attention. For tonight's game, we are playing on the body from the waist up only.

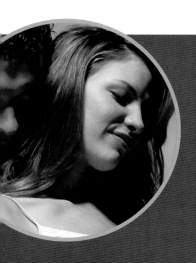

"I had no idea **how many desires I have** when taking time to 'see' my lover in this game. I'm used to thinking he was supposed to desire me and not so much the other way around. I love recognizing **how desirous and sensual I am,** and acting on my desires is powerful."

—CARMEN, AGE 45

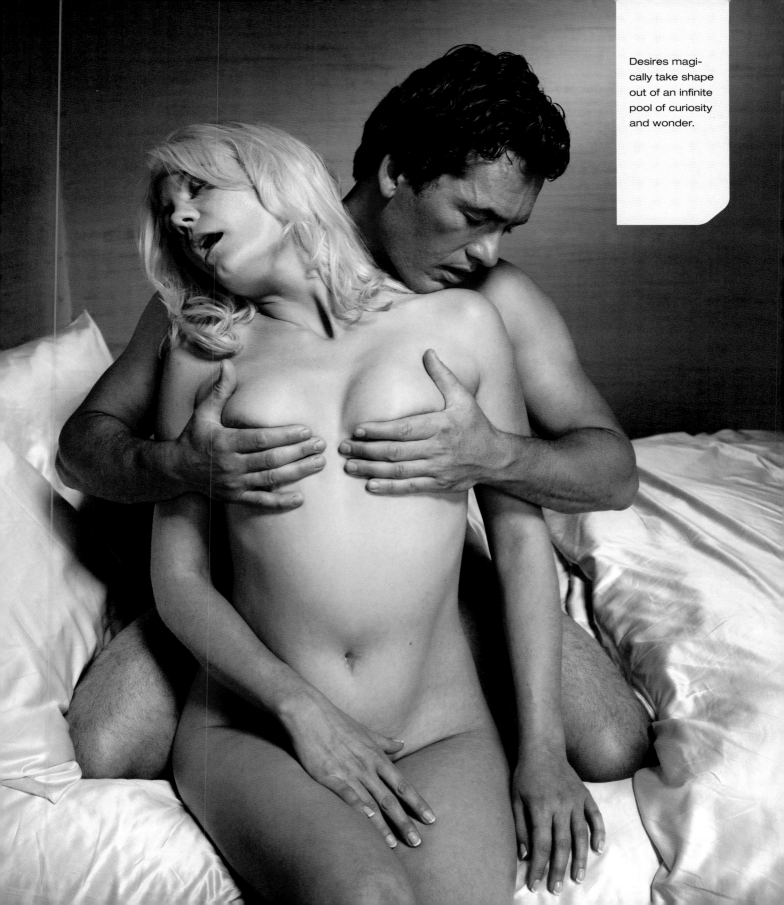

Desires magically take shape out of an infinite pool of curiosity and wonder.

Desire often feels like a tickle that wants to be scratched—a tingle that draws your attention to some specific place on another's body. Maybe you're drawn to the smooth skin on the curve of her neck where the light hits and you want to run the back of your hand along it. Perhaps you want to touch your partner's parted lips with your fingertips, run your fingers through her hair, smell the back of her neck, or lick a shoulder. Wait for something specific to show up for you; desire is not about making up anything or pretending. Settle back, survey the body softly with your relaxed curiosity, and allow desire to nudge at your fingertips.

Following your desire, ask your partner for permission to touch such as, "May I touch the dip at the base of your neck?" Your partner decides whether she wants that touch. She may say yes or no aloud or just nod her head. Touch until the desire has been sated, no longer, no less. Touch with interest, and when the interest stops, allow the next desire to emerge, and ask permission for the next touch.

Touch for your own satiety, trying not to anticipate what your partner may want. Desires magically take shape out of an infinite pool of curiosity and wonder. "May I touch the skin of your breasts and the cleavage along the lace of your nightgown?" Touch until the next desire tickles you. "May I play with your nipples through your nightgown?" Always wait for a positive response before touching, and touch only where you have been given permission.

Remember your partner's no is more about her than anything about you or your technique. Without judging your desires as wrong or her no as rejection, encourage your next desire to emerge. Out of the millions of possibilities on the body, you will discover your juicy common ground. At the end of three-minutes, bow in a Heart Salutation.

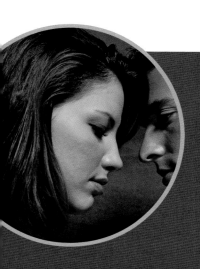

"My body felt so incredible, and he only touched my hair and shoulders. His voice was so sweet in asking. I felt the ultimate power rested with me even though I was in the passive, Yin role. I realized **I had the power to say yes or no** to touch on my body in each moment."

—VERONICA, AGE 29

ROUND 2: YOUR PARTNER ASKS TO TOUCH YOUR BODY (THREE MINUTES)

Change Yin/Yang roles so the woman is Yang, or active, and reset the timer for three minutes. Engage with your desires, let them play out on your partner's body. Ask for permission to explore him. Do not talk except for asking for permission and responding yes or no. Breathe deeply with your touching. At the end, take time to notice how it feels in your body to voice your desires, how it feels to have the final say over whether you are touched. Knowing the rules of safe touch is fundamental to feeling sexy.

ROUND 3: YOU ASK YOUR PARTNER TO TOUCH YOUR BODY (THREE MINUTES)

The next two rounds are similar to the first two, except you will be asking for touch on your own body versus your partner's body. Keep the same roles as last time, so the woman is Yang. Remember to keep this exercise to above the waist. Breathe and gaze together, becoming aware of your body. Tune into your body's sensations. Close your eyes if you'd like.

While breathing deeply, the woman focuses her attention solely on her body. Where do you want to be touched, nurtured, and attended to? When you feel a desire taking shape, ask for it, using words such as, "Please [rub, caress, kiss, or breathe on] my shoulders and upper arms." You are directing your partner's touch on your body. If he agrees, make sure he touches just the way you want it; fine-tune his touch to your liking. When you're ready for something else, ask for it.

Imagine you are Queen of the Universe and your sexy servant's sole desire is to "give it up" for you. Ask for the riches you deserve. When you've had enough of one thing, request whatever comes up next for you, such as, "Suck on my earlobes with soft puppy sounds."

Childlike, invite your heart's desires out to play. You may want to be held and rocked like a baby. Hear yourself ask for what you want. Play with the infinite field of possibilities. At the end of three minutes, observe how safe, sensual play enlivens your senses, curiosity, and joy. Take a few breaths to feel your body.

ROUND 4: YOUR PARTNER ASKS YOU TO TOUCH HIS BODY (THREE MINUTES)

For the last round, change Yin/Yang roles once more. Now the King of the Universe will ask his servant for the touch he desires on his body. This time the woman, in the serving position, is like a sexy kitten with the agility of an alley cat to "give" only what pleases you. As King, express to your "kitten" your heart's desire. Hear yourself ask for what you want on your body. This is about tuning into your needs, being attentive to you, and lapping it up like the family dog. You are not taking care of her. This is for you.

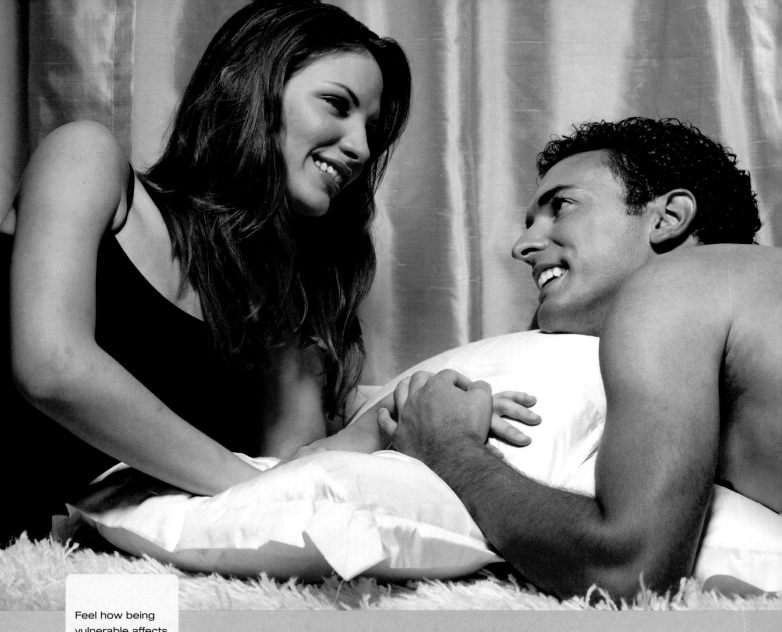

Feel how being
vulnerable affects
intimacy with your
partner.

Fantasies Are a Path to Wholeness

Fantasies come to you; you do not choose them. Often they express a unique blend of
unfulfilled desires from childhood, when you could not act on your natural sexual urges.
Growing up, you are faced with particular obstacles and challenges to overcome as a
sexual being in a sex-negative environment. Your collage of sexual fantasies helps you work
through, in dreamlike fashion, your journey to wholeness, integration, and health. Because
you are a unique "sexual snowflake," there are as many different sexualities as there are
people. Hence, judging someone's sexuality (or fantasies) becomes useless and accepting
one another a gesture of divine love.

Remember to ask permission before touching your partner's body to ensure safety in touch, which enlivens your senses, passion, and pleasure

End with a Heart Salutation and discussion (no more than two minutes each) of what the experience was like for each of you.

Erotic Exercise 3: **Expressing Sexual Fears, Fantasies, and Peak Experiences** [THIRTY MINUTES]

To build trust in a relationship, you must feel safe to talk openly about your sexuality and express what you want. Sex is the subject least talked about in most relationships, yet it's most important for love and intimacy. Hiding your sexual fears and turn-ons hinders trust and chokes creative sexual expression. In this exercise, you and your partner will take turns sharing sexual fears, fantasies, and peak experiences in order to get beyond shame and resistance that hinders your sexual expression.

SHARE SEXUAL FEARS

During the Opening Ritual, you release negative energy by naming it. Merely speaking a fear out loud diminishes it. Verbally sharing your sexual fears lessens their power over you. Decide who will speak first, and set the timer for five minutes. Similar to the automatic writing where your pen never stops moving, you will talk the entire time.

The listening partner asks, "What do you fear sexually?" Summarize a fear you have in a few sentences. A woman often fears, for example, that she will take too long to orgasm or that she won't come at all, that her body isn't attractive, or that you won't be able to tell her partner what she wants. A man often fears that his penis is too small, that he will come too quickly, that he won't be able to satisfy you, or that he will lose an erection.

After you state your fear in a brief sentence or two, give an example of the last time you remember the fear coming up and describe in detail what that was like for you. Keep defining your fears and giving specific examples until your time is up. If you stop talking, your partner may prompt you, "What is a sexual fear you have?"

The listener listens compassionately, without judgment or comment, and refrains from trying to reassure the speaker. Your listening is a powerful step in your partner's healing. You are a silent witness to your partner's naming and releasing of fears. At the end of five minutes of speaking, bring to a close your sharing, and bow in a Heart Salutation. The listener now thanks the speaker for their gifts of truth telling. Feel how being vulnerable affect intimacy with your partner. Share a Heart Salutation, reset the timer, and change roles.

SHARE SEXUAL FANTASIES

By sharing your sexual fantasies, you give your partner helpful information about your unique turn-ons. Besides being healthful, it can be hot to tread forbidden ground. Don't feel guilty or shamed about having fantasies: Break the silence, overturn past conditioning, and charge your sexuality with acceptance and approval. You may not choose to share all of your fantasies, but think of one you would be willing to tell your partner.

Reverse who starts first on this exercise, and set the timer for five minutes. When you speak, begin by telling a sexual fantasy. Remember to be detailed and descriptive: tell where you are and what time of day it is, give details about your partner(s), say what you are wearing, who's doing what to whom, etc. You are the storyteller, so relish in the juicy details of the scenario. If you stop speaking, your partner may say, "Tell me more about . . ." Everyone loves to hear a good story. When the timer sounds, conclude your fantasy. The listener then thanks the speaker. Share a Heart Salutation, reset the timer for five minutes, and changes roles to become the speaker.

SHARE PEAK SEXUAL EXPERIENCES

Sharing peak sexual experiences is a great opportunity to express what you love about making love. You surely have special sexual/sensual experiences you like to play back in your mind. As a couple, you may want to pick an experience from your shared lovemaking background, unless both of you feel secure enough to open it up to past experiences.

Decide who will share first. Set the timer for five minutes and pick a past peak sexual experience you are willing to share with your partner. Describe in detail the scenario, where you are, how it started, how it progressed, etc. Include what made it so special and what you were feeling. Keep talking for the whole time. The listener should not comment on your peak experience, only prompt you for more detail if necessary. At the end, he will thank you for sharing and end with a Heart Salutation. Can you appreciate your partner's vulnerability in sharing? Reset the timer for five minutes, and change roles. Do not think your peak sexual experience has to be anything like your partner's. It's yours.

Erotic Exercise 4: Making Sensual Requests That Get Results [TEN MINUTES]

You may not express what you want 100 percent of the time while in the moment because you think you will sound needy or demanding. Yet there is a way to make requests that invite heartfelt compliance. In the Three-Step Request, (1) validate your partner, (2) give him one "doable" thing to do, and (3) appreciate him for it.

- **Validate your partner.** Tell him something he is doing right now or in general that you like about him.

- **Ask for one, clear, doable thing that you want from your partner.** Do not ask for two things, and do not be vague.

- **Appreciate your partner for honoring your request.**

Learning this Three-Step Request—validating, asking, and honoring your partner—will encourage you to express more of your desires, because the process is so enjoyable. This exercise is also called the Sandwich Request, because you express something you like about your partner (top piece of bread), you ask for what you want (the middle "jelly" layer), and you appreciate him for giving it to you (the bottom bread). Here are a few examples:

- "Your touch is gorgeous. Please move more slowly. Oh, yes, that's great."

- "I love the pressure of your stroke. Could you try using the whole hand and forearm? You got it, wonderful!"

- "Your touch is deliciously slow. I'd like it lighter too. Even lighter. Oh, yes, that's dreamy."

- "It's heaven getting massaged by you. My feet want your attention, too. Oh, thank you."

With your partner, practice making at least three Sandwich Requests back and forth. Help your partner fine-tune his requests, especially if he does not validate you at the beginning or appreciate you at the end enough, or if a request is not clear, or if he asks for more than one thing. Three-Step Requests work well on all people and all occasions. Try them out on children, friends, bosses, and a spouse you'd like to have out the garbage.

Erotic Exercise 5: Front Body Caresses with Three-Step Requests   [FIFTY MINUTES]

You will be giving and receiving from your partner a twenty-minute front Body Caress and practicing Sandwich Requests. The front body is more sensitive than the back body, and you may feel more vulnerable and exposed with your underbelly up, as your genitals and breasts are showing. This exercise will especially challenge your adherence to the Rules for Touching (page 39), such as tuning into your sensations, focusing on your pleasure in touching, and letting go of the need to go anyplace with the caress.

Decide who will receive first, and undress to whatever level feels comfortable for you in the moment. Lie face-up on a bed or soft pad with pillows. Make sure you are warm enough. Turn up the music. The toucher (in this case, the woman) collects feathers, furs, a scent mister, a silk scarf, and cornstarch, and sets the timer for twenty minutes. Kneeling by your partner's left side, put your left hand over his or her abdomen and your right over his heart. Come into the body by Soul Gazing and Ocean Breathing.

Ask for permission to include the genitals (and breasts for a woman) in a frontal caress if you desire to touch them. Asking for permission for genital touch is always respectful. Even with permission, do not focus on them; rather, include them casually as you honor the whole body with caressing. Except for any sensual request from the touchee, the massage is nonverbal.

During this frontal caress, the receiver will make several Three-Step Requests of the giver, just for practice, if nothing else. The giver begins by gently rocking the body from the heart/abdomen hold. Then trace lightly from the heart down both arms and back, down the torso, legs, and feet with long, slow, soft strokes covering the whole front body as an introduction to the caress. Breathe deeply, modeling a breath that slows the chatter of the mind. Follow the sound of your breath, sighing on the exhale to pull yourself into the present moment.

Remind him to surrender deeper into the body with each exhale and simply enjoy every sensation. There is no destination, just the journey. He doesn't have to become hard or aroused, though it's fine if it happens. Float a silk scarf over his body several times, letting the fringe tickle his inner thighs. Drape the scarf over his torso, and lightly play with his nipples and genitals through the silky fabric. Slip a rabbit fur glove between each toe and up the sides of his body and underarms. With a peacock feather, tease his earlobes, face, and lips.

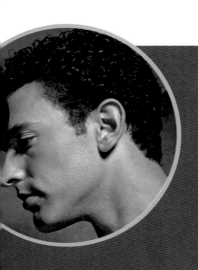

"I loved it when Lindsey told me this front caress was just for me and there was nothing I had to do [get hard] and no place I had to go [get aroused]. She wanted me to **enjoy the touch and that's all.** I realized how often I think I have to initiate and go somewhere in sex. This is new and very helpful for me."

—JIM, AGE 27

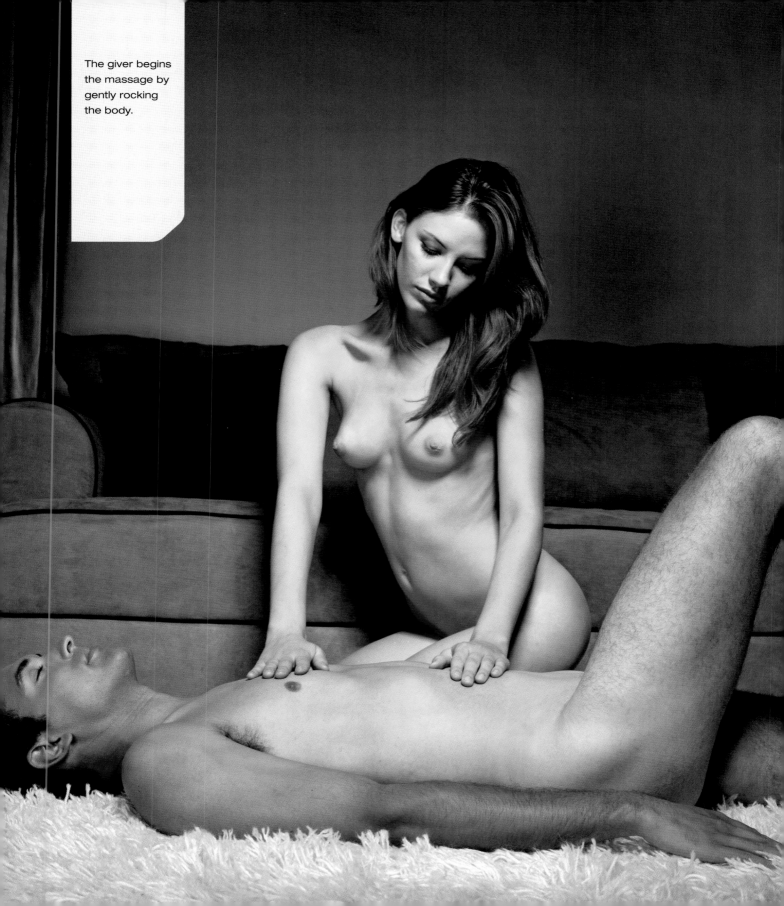

The giver begins
the massage by
gently rocking
the body.

Halfway through, if your touchee has not made any Three-Step Requests yet, remind him or her to make one. How might you fine-tune your touching for his pleasure? In about five minutes, ask your receiver to make a second Three-Step Request. This is good practice. Did your partner validate you first, and then ask for one thing clearly, remembering to appreciate you after you gave it to him?

Let each stoke flow into the next in a seamless dance, the last stroke transitioning to the next. End the caress with the same slow, sweeping, full-body stokes and gentle heart/abdomen (or genital) rocking as you began. Take a few moments in silence to enjoy erotic pleasure of giving and receiving heartfelt touch. Appreciate your journey into timeless and treasured moments exploring the body erotic. End in a Heart Salutation, reset the timer for twenty minutes, and change roles.

Erotic Exercise 6: Closing Ritual   [TEN MINUTES]

In closing this Erotic Night on expressing desires, reread your Ecstasy Journal entries on What Turns Me On Romantically and What Turns Me On Sexually. Underline five things in each entry that you are willing to share with your partner at this time. Read them aloud to each other. If you choose not to share from your journal, that's fine, too. In place of sharing from the journal, do the following exercise:

Sit opposite one another. Set the timer for two minutes, and ask your partner, "How do you like to be touched?" Let your partner talk for the total two minutes while you listen for essence without commenting. At the end of two minutes, exchange roles. Now switch again, set the timer for two minutes, and ask your partner, "How do you like to be teased?" At the end of two minutes, exchange roles.

Looking Ahead

• Make sensual Three-Step Requests of each other in the coming days.

• Notice how often you express your desires versus deny them in the coming days. Write in your Ecstasy Journal on this subject if you'd like.

• Read Erotic Night Four several days before it takes place.

Close the evening by performing the same simple ritual or gesture as you have done on previous Erotic Nights. Delay regular conversation until the ceremonial ending of the evening is complete by cleaning up and blowing out the candles together. Leave the Sensual Space and remember your promises of keeping what happens in that space confidential and of containing erotic energy without intercourse the rest of the night.

Erotic Recap

- Opening Ritual: *thirty minutes*
- Playing the Three-Minute Game: Asking for What You Want: *fifteen minutes*
- Expressing Sexual Fears, Fantasies, and Peak Experiences: *thirty minutes*
- Making Sensual Requests That Get Results: *ten minutes*
- Front Body Caresses with Three-Step Requests: *fifty minutes*
- Closing Ritual: *ten minutes*

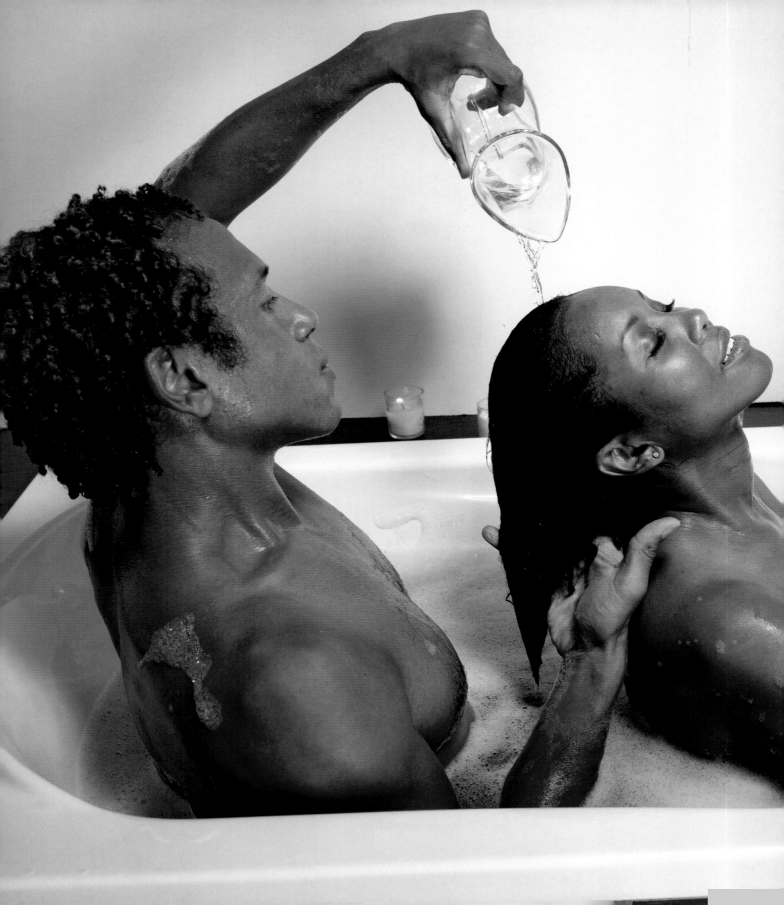

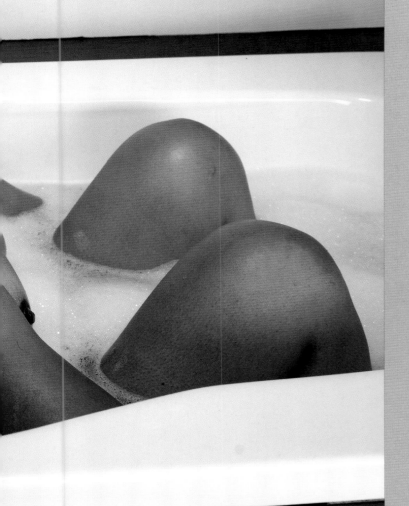

EROTIC NIGHT
FOUR

Appreciating Your Partner with Body-Honoring Rituals

During the previous Erotic Night, you learned how expressing your desires keeps your body alive and your relationships fresh. Expressing desires is invigorating in itself, independent of the outcome or how others respond to them. In the Three-Minute Game, by asking permission before you touched your partner, you crafted safe agreements that enhanced sensuality. On previous nights, you practiced making Three-Step Requests, which validate, instruct, and honor your partner.

Tonight, you will approve and appreciate your partner as a unique sensual/sexual being with body-honoring rituals. When you feel appreciated rather than judged by your partner, you feel safe, playful, and sexy. A backdrop of expressing appreciation sets the stage for electric and passionate sex.

Erotic Exercise 1: Opening Ritual [THIRTY MINUTES]

On the day of your Erotic Night, eat lightly, exercise, drink lots of water, and review this night/chapter. Show up with time to spare, comfortably clothed, with a clean mouth and body. In a ceremonial fashion, prepare your Sensual Space together with soft romantic lighting and music.

1. **Sit opposite each other and set the timer for each of your two-minute Weather Reports, including Come Cleans,** which follow the format "I noticed . . . I felt . . . I need . . . and I request." Remember to be concise and thank your partner for Come Cleans without any additional comments. Appreciate how this Opening Ritual lets you put away the happenings of the day and any matter that may distract you from being present, attentive, and sensual with your partner for the rest of the evening.

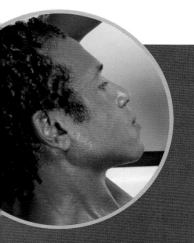

"The ritual of **preparing the space together** acts like a bridge for me. With each candle I light I leave behind my ordinary, busy day, where I live in my head, and enter a world of slowness,

2. **Create sacred space by clearing away negativity and calling in positive qualities to sanctify your room.** By naming that which you wish to rid or attract, you transform the mundane into the sacred. Where you put your attention, energy flows. Set the tone for the evening by speaking your intention in positive language such as, "I intend my every word and touch to come from my heart," or "I intend to soften and enjoy my body."

3. **Come into the body with Ocean Breathing for five minutes.** Set the timer. Relax into a slower, deeper breath as you follow the breath in and out with all your attention. Sigh softly on the exhale through a loose throat and jaw. Become aware of how softening the jaw relates to opening the pelvic region to increased blood flow and sensation. While Soul Gazing into each other's eyes, let your breath to fall into a shared pattern. Allow a softness to come over you, a blurred space between your beings, a place of non-judgment and peace. Fall freely in and out of trance states.

4. **Play four rounds of the Three-Minute Game that you played on Erotic Night Three.** Enjoy expressing just how you desire to touch your partner and be pleasured by your partner. Set the timer for three minutes for each of the following rounds: (1) you asking for permission to touch your partner's body, (2) your partner asking for permission to touch your body, (3) you asking for your partner to touch your body how you desire, and (4) your partner asking you to touch his or her body how he or she desires. End in a Heart Salutation.

Feel the solid ground created for erotic encounters by expressing desires, asking for permission to touch another, being responsible to express your own boundaries, and letting go of any outcome. These are guideposts pointing to rapturous sex.

dropping down into my body. **I savor sinking into body time and relishing the joy of shared intimacy** with my partner."

—DAMION, AGE 35

Erotic Exercise 2: **Talking Genitals**   [THIRTY MINUTES]

In this exercise, give your genitals a chance to speak, and you listen to the wisdom that per-colates up from your "down under." You may seldom tap into this natural body, but by giving voice to your genitals and hearing their story, you'll uncover another perspective. Hearing details of your partner's sexual story translates into deeper respect, closeness, and juicy sex.

From the moment you were born, your genitals colored the story of who you are. You learned early how little boys and little girls are different from each other. You received messages from your parents, teachers, and community about being male or female. You learned quickly how you were supposed to act, dress, and talk; what you were supposed to like; and how you were supposed to feel about the opposite sex.

You may also have internalized the cultural silence and shame around your genitals. You learned not to touch your "private parts" (even though it felt good), and not to ask questions or talk about "down there." I hadn't even heard of the word "clitoris" until I got to college.

SPEAK AS IF YOU ARE YOUR PENIS (OR VULVA)

In this exercise, have fun speaking as your penis or vulva and discover just how articulate, funny, and wise this gorgeous part of you is. Decide who will share first (we'll use the man in this case), set the timer for fifteen minutes, sit comfortably with your back supported and legs open, and bare your genitals if you feel brave, though it's not necessary.

Start speaking as if you were your penis, and talk about your life using "I" statements such as, "I remember when [speaker's name] was a child and first discovered and played with me . . . I remember him showing me off to so and so . . . One day he got caught play-ing with me and such and such happened . . . I remember the messages he heard about me from parents and teachers, and they made me feel . . . I remember when he got a girl-

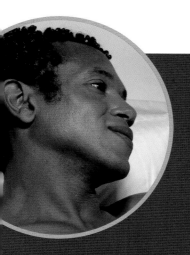

"I never realized what **a sense of humor my penis has.** He told me to quit treating him like an old married couple and that he was bored and I'd better bring some variety into his life!"

—WILL, AGE 47

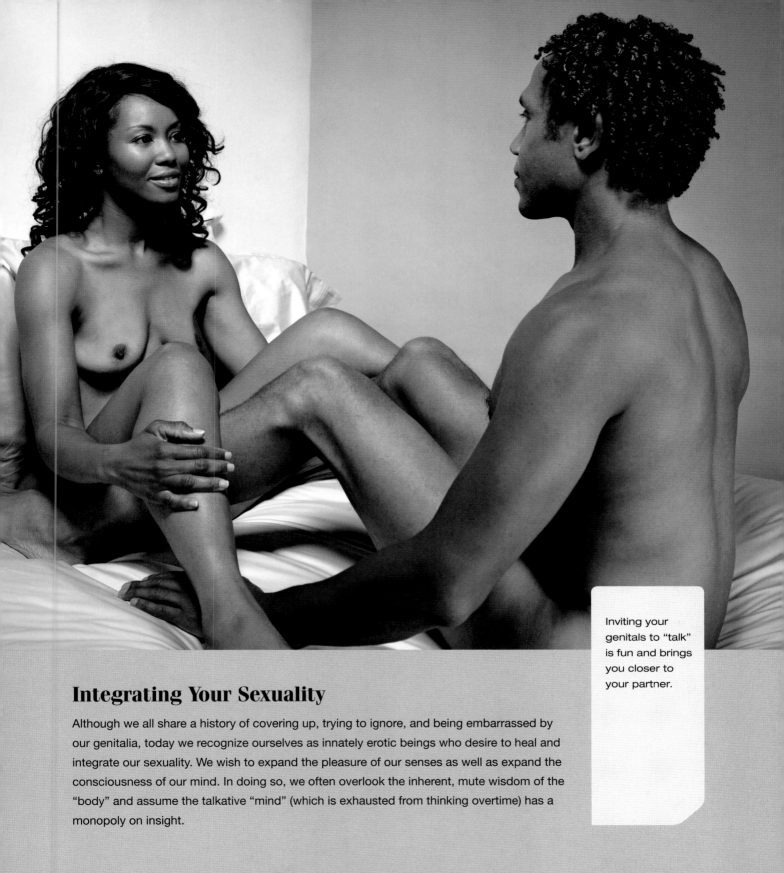

Inviting your genitals to "talk" is fun and brings you closer to your partner.

Integrating Your Sexuality

Although we all share a history of covering up, trying to ignore, and being embarrassed by our genitalia, today we recognize ourselves as innately erotic beings who desire to heal and integrate our sexuality. We wish to expand the pleasure of our senses as well as expand the consciousness of our mind. In doing so, we often overlook the inherent, mute wisdom of the "body" and assume the talkative "mind" (which is exhausted from thinking overtime) has a monopoly on insight.

friend, I felt . . . With his first kisses, I felt . . . first wet dream . . . first masturbation . . . first intercourse . . .," and so on.

While your genitals do the talking, you (and your partner) are listening for essence. Let your penis extol, "The best part of my life now is . . . I'm afraid, though, about . . . My master does [or doesn't] listen to me in this way . . ." End the talk with this important statement, "An important and wise message I have to say is . . ." As the timer sounds, give your penis a Heart Salutation and thank him for sharing his wisdom with you and being so articulate. You may decide to let him know you will check in more often if it's agreeable to the both of you.

Reset the timer for fifteen minutes, and now the woman will let her vulva do the talking. Sit opposite your partner with legs gently falling apart; bare your genitals if it's comfortable for you. Talk about many of the same experiences as suggested for the man by changing the gender pronouns in the preceding paragraph. Include some particular female talk such as, "Here's what I thought upon learning about where babies come from . . . During my first menstrual period, I felt . . . During my first pregnancy, I felt . . . When I had an abortion, I felt . . . When I gave birth, I felt . . ."

Let your vulva express, "What I enjoy most now is . . . What I'm most afraid of is . . . How I could be more appreciated is . . ." And end with, "The important wisdom I have to share with you tonight is . . ." Thank your vulva for being so expressive, and give her a Heart Salutation. Would she like you to check in more often? Much wisdom is stored in the body, accessible only if you are attentive. Has your partner, by revealing and being vulnerable, touched a shared humanity with you? If you have touched your genitals during this exercise, wash your hands.

Erotic Exercise 3: **Reflecting on Body Image**
[THIRTY MINUTES]

You likely have issues with your body. You may feel you are too skinny, too fat, too bumpy, or too this or that. Because every model you see in the media has a perfect body, you may wonder what happened to you. Body image is important in sex. You carry what you think about your body into your relationships, and negative feelings can numb and hamper your sexual sensations. Cultivating a supportive attitude toward your maturing, imperfect body graces life with softness, compassion, and sensuality.

In this exercise, look and comment on your body with honesty and an eye for self-love and acceptance. For the Body Image Exercise, one partner bravely steps into the active role (in this case the woman).

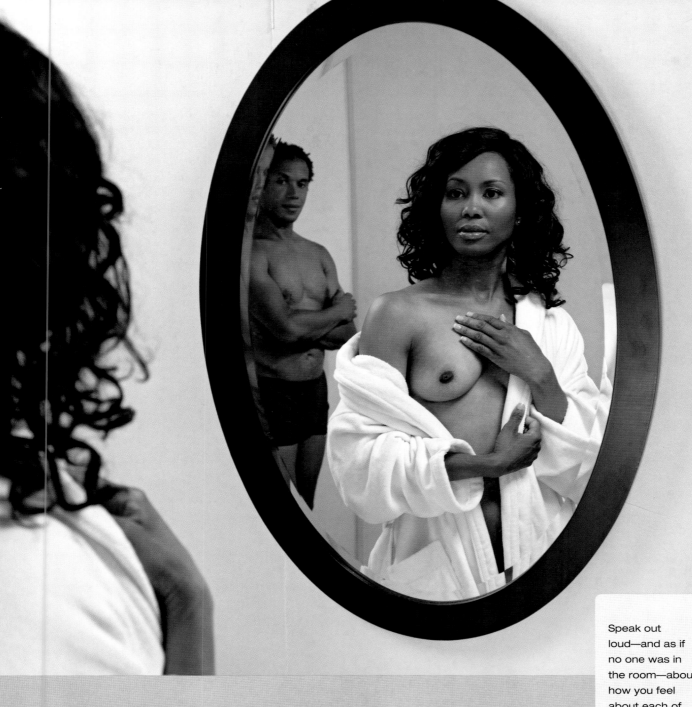

Speak out loud—and as if no one was in the room—about how you feel about each of your body parts.

An Earthly Temple

Your body is no less than the earthly temple of your thoughts, emotions, and spirit. In this body, you see reflected back to you all the pain, excitement, sorrow, and joy of every moment you have lived. Your body, for better or for worse, is your home for every experience you have lived and have yet to live. Self-love and appreciation is a stepping-stone to partner love and appreciation. Self-acceptance rather than self-criticism is the pathway to great sex.

1. **Set the timer for fifteen minutes, and stand naked, or with as little clothing as is comfortable, in front of a full-length mirror.** Ask your partner to make himself comfortable sitting on the floor with pillows behind you; he is a silent, attentive, and supportive witness to your exploration and monologue.

2. **Close your eyes.** Breathing deeply and slowly, focus attention onto your body.

3. **Open your eyes when you're ready, and begin surveying your body from head to toe in the mirror.** Even though your partner is present, this exercise is for you. With a reverent attitude, begin speaking out loud to yourself, as if no one else were in the room, about how you feel about each body part, starting at the head and ending with your toes.

4. **Survey your body.** What do you think about your hair? What do you like or not like about your forehead, eyes, nose, mouth, and face? Be honest in your verbal commentary, voicing compliments as well as your reservations. Look at your shoulders, chest, abdomen, and genitals. Talk aloud; use a stream of consciousness to relay your thoughts and feelings about each body part. Laugh, smile, and tell a story if it pops up.

5. **Feel free to touch yourself and stay looking at a part until any charge dissipates before moving on.** Turn around to look at your back and butt in the mirror. How do you feel about them? Include your anus, usually over-shamed and underappreciated in most of us. Continue down your body to your thighs, legs, feet, and toes. Can you regard your scars, wrinkles, moles, and imperfections as proud testaments of your experience and wisdom?

6. **At the end, breathe and close your eyes.** Take time to appreciate how vulnerable you may feel exposing your true feelings about your body in front of your partner. Has such an exercise encouraged you to accept and appreciate your body more? How may it free up your loving? End with a Heart Salutation.

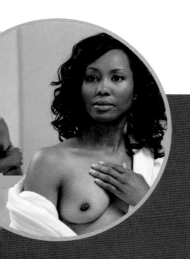

"I thought the Body Image Exercise would be difficult because **I'm so critical about my body**. Yet in the mirror, I saw past all its imperfections; **I sensed how much joy my body has**

As the silent partner, you may have noticed parts of her body that were left out or underappreciated. Take note, as these will need your extra loving care. Thank your partner, recognizing her courageous risk-taking by exposing her true feelings about her body. Reset the timer for fifteen minutes, and trade roles.

Erotic Exercise 4: **Anointing Your Partner with Sacred Oil**   [FORTY MINUTES]

In this luscious body ritual, you will take turns acting as a Shamanic Priest or Priestess. You will ceremonially bless with sacred oil your partner's body, anointing then massaging while expressing aloud appreciation for each body part from feet to head. Appreciation heals and tunes your body for heightened sensation and joy in sex.

As the active partner, pour oil into a special bowl, and set the timer for twenty minutes while the woman lies comfortably on a bed or mat with pillows, preferably nude. Sit or kneel at her left (heart) side, and place one hand over her heart and the other over her abdomen (or genitals with permission). Come into the body by Soul Gazing and Ocean Breathing together. Bless the oil in the bowl by waving your hand over it while you state your intention for this ritual, using words such as, "I intend to honor my beloved's body," or, "I intend to bless my partner with an open, loving heart." The receiver states her intention for receiving your blessings on her body. She may intend to "open my body to greater love" or "appreciate my body" or "be aware of my divine nature."

Starting at the feet, dip into the sacred oil (now that is it imbued with your blessings) and, as you anoint each foot with oil, say, "I anoint these feet as the vehicle of your spirit." After the anointment, massage while giving praises to her feet such as, "These feet have carried you to me. They have walked many miles taking care of our children and helping our families and community. These lovely feet have traveled to distant lands on vacations with me. They have wrapped around my torso in joyous lovemaking." End with a blessing, "I bless and honor these feet with love."

brought my lover—and me. I've decided to make a new friend—my body—and share it more often with more joy."

—VALERIE, AGE 34

Move up to the legs, and repeat anointing, massaging, and blessing the legs. Dip into your oil and say, "I anoint these legs as a vehicle of your spirit." Continue adoring, complimenting, and giving gratitude for these legs alound in your own words. Be generous, compassionate, sexy, and turned on. End with a blessing such as, "I bless and honor these legs with love." Anoint her thighs using the same Three-Step Appreciation. Thighs are synonymous with strength, fluidity, and action.

Ask for permission to lay a hand over her genitals. She may prefer to lay your hand over hers on top of her genitals. Place your other hand over her abdomen, a move that makes one feel protected and secure. Say, "I anoint this beautiful [flower, jewel, garden of

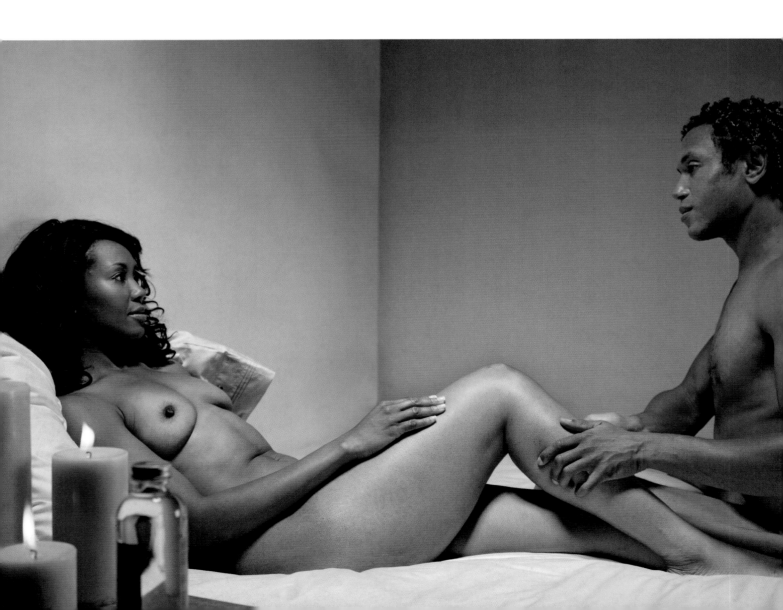

pleasure, or however you may choose to name her genitals] as a vehicle of your spirit." In luscious but authentic words, describe the beauty, pleasure, and delight you relish from this gorgeous part of her. Keep your hands still except for perhaps a small, gentle vibration while speaking. End with, "I bless and honor this orchid flower with love."

Anoint the abdomen, center of digesting food and experiences. Anoint the breasts (heart center of love and playfulness), the arms (holding and cherishing), hands (creativity), shoulders (strength and work), and head (intuition and intellect). Anoint, massage while giving praises, and end with a blessing, "I bless and honor . . ." You are the ceremonial priest giving her body a blessing she has probably never had before. Ritualistically attend to her and appreciate each part. Plan your time so you may bless the whole body without rushing.

After you blessed the entire body, again rest a hand over her heart and the other over her genitals. Connecting these two centers through your touch completes the sacred marriage of two powerful and complementary body centers—love from the heart and power from the root (genitals). Breathe together, and take a moment to notice how giving and receiving appreciation feels in the body.

In closing, inhale deeply together, and listen as the receiver finishes this sentence aloud while exhaling, "I am aware . . ." What is one thing you notice or observe in the present moment? Do not work at your answer or think about your response; there is no right answer. Just state one thing you are aware of, and when you run out of breath, stop talking. Again inhale deeply together, and this time the giver finishes the sentence while exhaling, "I am aware . . ." Again, respond only one breath's worth. The truth is short. We often get heady and go into a thinking space when we go on. Exchange a Heart Salutation, reset the timer for twenty minutes, and switch roles.

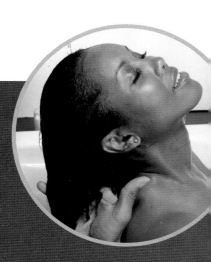

"I loved him so much after he **anointed my body with oil and touch**; we went deeper into the heart of our loving."

—NATALIA, AGE 45

Erotic Exercise 5: The Tantric Kiss with the Sexual Breath and the Love Pump [TWENTY MINUTES]

In Tantra, the pelvic floor muscle is referred to as the Love Pump, and by strengthening it you will increase pleasurable sensations in your sex organs as well as prolong and strengthen your orgasms and erections. You can learn how to exercise this most important muscle, and how to pulse it during lovemaking to move energy up the spine to intensify sexual sensations and connection. Tonight we will add Love Pump pulses to Sexual Breathing and the Tantric Kiss. These techniques cultivate potent sexual energy in the body and deepen erotic trance states.

TECHNIQUE #1: LOVE PUMP

To find your pubococcygeal (or PC muscle), flex the muscle you use to stop a stream of urine while peeing. Or imagine sitting down on hot sand at the beach and quickly pulling up on your pelvic floor to keep from burning. This flexing is also known as the Kegel exercise. Your PC muscle is the muscle that involuntarily pulses during orgasm. Try flexing it a few times now, paying special attention to keep your butt, abdomen, and thigh muscles soft and relaxed. These are PC Pulses.

Usually weak, this muscle responds quickly to exercise, and if you commit to daily pulses of your PC, you will notice a difference with stronger and longer orgasms within a couple of weeks. This Love Pump is your ticket to healthy sex organs, longevity, multi-orgasms for men, and female ejaculation (if you choose). A toned PC muscle in women can erotically milk the penis during penetration sex.

After several pulses, you may notice a tingling sensation in your genitals. Enjoy the wakeup call. A good starting PC exercise regimen is twenty pulses each morning, noon, and night. Pull up on the pelvic floor for the count "one potato, two potato" and then completely release all tension for the same count "one potato, two potato." Make sure you totally relax between each pulse to release all tension or even push out a little. When I see the bodybuilders work out in the gym, I wonder if they really know the most important muscle to exercise! Start daily toning of you Love Pump for potent, multi-orgasmic loving.

TECHNIQUE #2: THE SEXUAL BREATH

The Sexual Breath elongates Ocean Breathing by adding a hold to the top and bottom of each inhale and exhale. With this breath, you feel an increased streaming and pulsing of natural erotic energy in the body. High Sex or Tantra has much to say about breathing. This Sexual Breath is only one of hundreds of ways to manipulate the four-part breath formula for erotic embodiment.

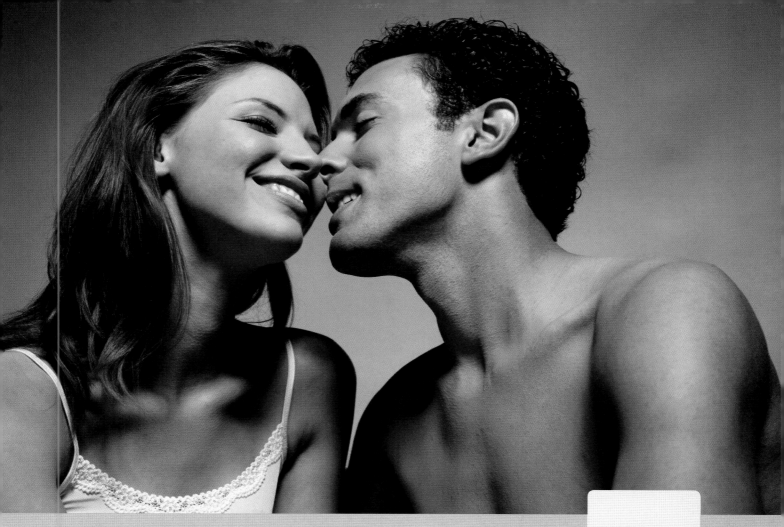

The Tantric Kiss

The Tantric Kiss is an ancient circular exchange of essence between the male/female prin-
cipals, or Yin/Yang. In Tantra, Shiva, male god of consciousness, and Shakti, female god-
dess of energy and light, blend their essences in a joyful, playful dance of love that spawns
all creation. The woman in this kiss imagines on her exhale sending her heart energy into
the man's heart. On her inhale, she imagines receiving root energy from the man's *lingam*
(penis) in through her *yoni* (vagina). The man imagines on his exhale sending root energy out
through his *lingam* into the woman's *yoni*. On his inhale, he imagines taking in heart energy
from the woman's heart. In Tantric wisdom, the man is strong in the root, and the woman
is strong in the heart. With this breath and kiss exchange, partners takes in what they need
and give out their strength. Each breath perfectly balances each partner. Tantric breathing
and kissing heals, strengthens, and enlightens. You become balanced, enriched, and enliv-
ened by this breath of life.

The Tantric Kiss
is your gateway
to whole-body
and energy
orgasms.

Practice the sexual breath by counting to five (approximately five seconds) on each of the following four aspects of the breath: (1) intake, (2) hold at top of the breath, (3) exhale, and (4) hold at bottom of the breath. According to Tantric wisdom, slowing the intake breath increases the body's spirit (fire), pausing at the top opens the body to inspiration (air), breathing out releases the body's emotional aspect (water), and holding at the bottom grounds the body (earth).

TECHNIQUE #3: THE SEXUAL BREATH WITH THE LOVE PUMP

Set the timer for five minutes, and sit opposite each other and in a loose yab-yum position, the woman's legs over the man's and your hands resting on each other's legs. Gaze and breathe together. Begin extending your breathing by silently counting to five on each of the four aspects of the breath—inhale, pause, exhale, pause. Watch your partner's breathing, and synchronize your rhythm.

After a couple of minutes, when this four-part rhythm feels natural, add PC Pulses to your pauses after the inhale and exhale. Contract your Love Pump for "one potato, two potato," then release it completely for "one potato, two potato." Try a second contraction if you like. Continue breathing in sync with pauses, and add PC Pulses to the pauses at the top and bottom of each breath. If your Love Pump tires, that's okay—just pause without contracting.

TECHNIQUE #4: THE TANTRIC KISS WITH THE SEXUAL BREATH

Brush your teeth again or take a breath mint before this intimate breath exercise with your partner. You will practice kissing your partner with the techniques of the Sexual Breath, alternating the Sexual Breath, and then adding PC Pulses. In the Tantric Kiss, you will be building erotic body skills you may use in your lovemaking. Set the timer for seven minutes. The woman sits on the man's lap, her head above his in the classic yab-yum Tantric position. Both of you touch your feet together behind each other's back if you are flexible enough. Loosely put your lips together with air space around them so there is no suction. Begin breathing the five-count Sexual Breath together. Your eyes may be open or closed.

TECHNIQUE #5: THE TANTRIC KISS WITH ALTERNATE SEXUAL BREATHING

After a couple of minutes, the man will change his breathing so he is inhaling when the woman exhales. You are breathing in and out at opposite times now, keeping the pauses at the top and bottom of the breath. You are literally breathing in the essence of the other and giving back to them your essence. Breathe like this for several minutes.

TECHNIQUE #6: THE TANTRIC KISS WITH ALTERNATING BREATHING AND THE LOVE PUMP EXERCISE

After the alternate breathing is established, add PC Pulses to any pause when you so desire, not particularly each time. Do not worry about how many or how long your pulses are. Let go of counting for now. Relax into a shared rhythm, adding your PC Pulses when you feel inclined. Pace yourself. Don't overdo PC work in the beginning. This small muscle tires easily, and it's better to work it up gradually. Can you envision the energy moving up the spine from the genitals by the Love Pump?

Allow yourself to give and take of the ancient air, the eternal dance of the masculine and feminine. Enjoy your role as current players in this timeless ritual of blending the male and female essences. Invite trance states to carry you past the personalities involved, past separateness, and to merge formless into the sea of cosmic union. This is your true state as much as any other. Own it. Be it. Great sex is your birthright. You are wired for it.

If it seems like a lot to remember, simply enjoy the breath together. If you get lost, fine—smile and get back together. You're putting a lot of pieces together, and it will take practice—like adding a couple of minutes of kiss to the Daily Erotic Ritual from time to time. With practice, you will fall effortlessly into the grace of this kiss, which also is the gateway to whole-body and energy orgasms.

Erotic Exercise 6: Closing Ritual

Tonight, you have listened to wisdom from your Talking Genitals, viewed your body in the mirror with compassion, received body blessings from your beloved, and shared the Tantric Kiss with new techniques for expanded bliss. You were heard, seen, touched, and kissed by your partner with deep attention and sacred intention. Notice how your body feels.

In closing, ask your partner two questions: "How can I support you in becoming the person you want to be?" and, "What risks might you want to take, and how can I support you in them?" Set the timer for five minutes for his or her response to these questions. If you choose to support your partner in one or more of the ways she suggests, signify in some way your willingness. Reset the timer and change roles.

Looking Ahead

Close your ceremonial evening with your ritual ending. This familiar saying or gesture gives closure to the evening, just as the creating of sacred space gave a beginning. In this manner, the night is contained between these two rituals. Refrain from ordinary conversation until you blow out the candles and leave the Sensual Space. Remember to honor your initial agreements to keep what happens in the Sensual Space sacred. Before bringing up the events or sharings from this evening, remember to ask for permission first. And remember your agreement to refrain from orgasmic release or penetration sex on this and all Erotic Nights.

Prepare for the next Erotic Night by shopping that same day for food treats and other sensual surprises to give your partner during a Blindfolded Ceremony of Sensual Delights (see Erotic Night Five before shopping). Come with the food items in a paper bag so they remain a surprise for your partner. Collect a few essential oils and perhaps a new prop for sensual touching (consider visiting a sex shop). Also bring your partner a small wrapped gift to present during the next Erotic Night's opening ceremony.

Read Erotic Night Five a few days before it takes place.

Erotic Recap

- Opening Ritual: *thirty minutes*

- Talking Genitals: *thirty minutes*

- Reflecting on Body Image: *thirty minutes*

- Anointing Your Partner with Sacred Oil: *forty minutes*

- The Tantric Kiss with the Sexual Breath and the Love Pump: *twenty minutes*

- Closing Ritual: *ten minutes*

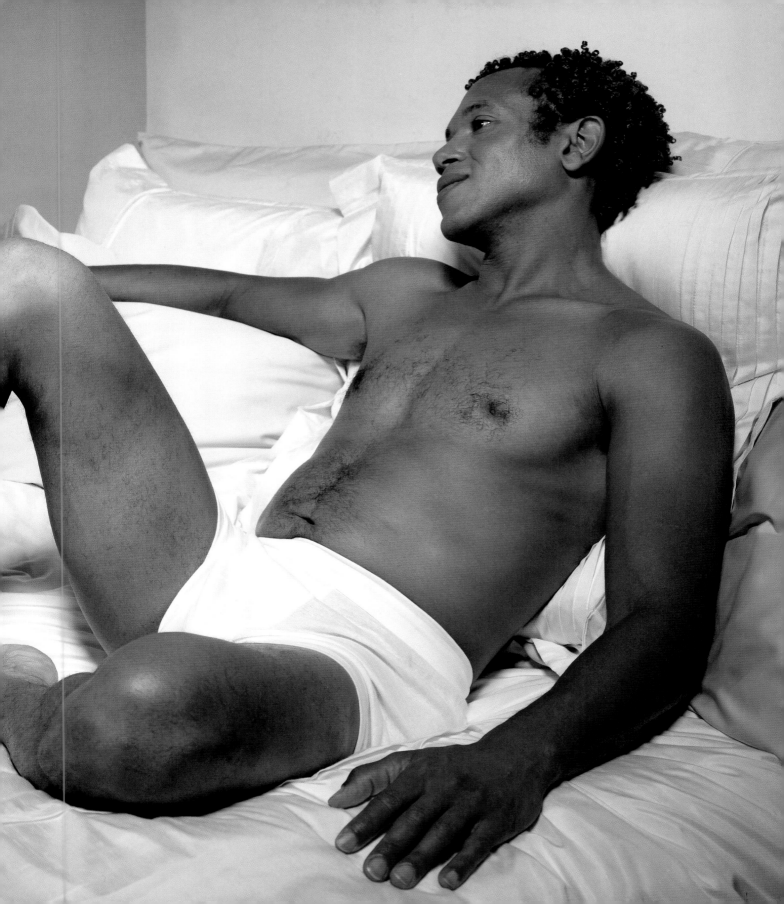

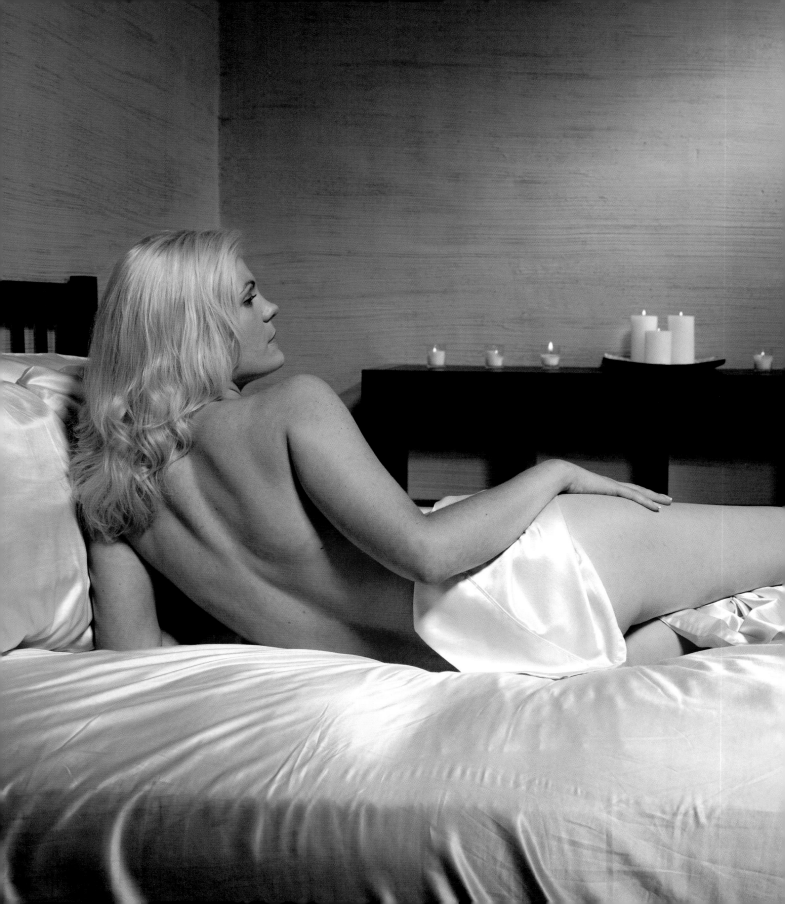

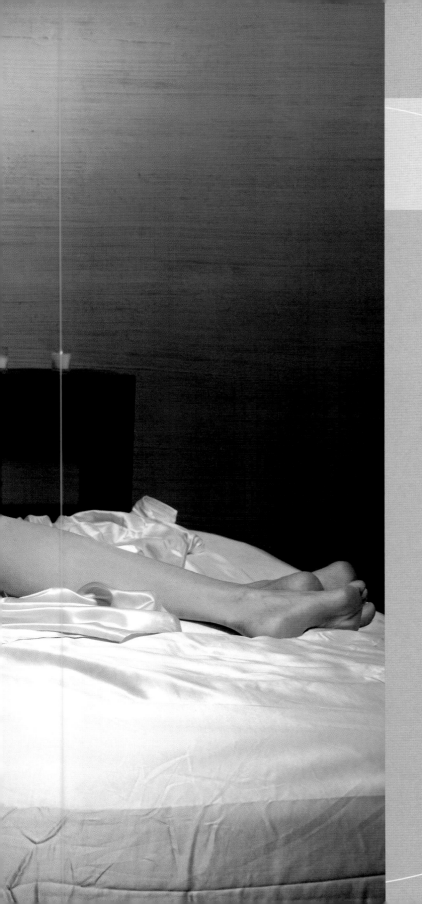

EROTIC NIGHT
FIVE

Honoring
the Body Erotic

During the previous Erotic Night, you listened to your genitals speak, shared your feelings about your body, received your partner's body blessings, and practiced the PC Pulses with the Tantric Kiss as a pathway to extended erotic trance and orgasms.

Tonight, you will sensually delight your partner with a Blindfolded Ceremony of Sensual Delights. When you awaken, tease, and heighten the body's senses, you increase sensual awareness during lovemaking. And tonight, you will also self-pleasure your genitals while your partner silently watches. It's hot to see your lover turned on, and it's reassuring to remember that you are in charge of your own turn-on. Sharing masturbation can make this normal and natural act a positive and arousing part of partner sexuality.

Erotic Exercise 1: Opening Ritual [TWENTY MINUTES]

For this Erotic Night, pay attention, tell the truth, and stay open to the outcome. Invite yourself to be present tonight and know that what you put into this evening is what you will get out of it. You decide how much you take away from this experience by how much you give of yourself. To begin, take the following steps:

1. **Be aware the day of your date to be kind to your body.** Eat lightly, get exercise, and drink lots of water. Our body, like a finely tuned vehicle, runs better with good fuel and good care. Be leisurely in your grooming preparations, and show up with time to spare. Keep your Sensual Delight items hidden from you partner in order to create suspense and surprise—also characteristics for great sex. Have your gift ready to present to your partner.

2. **Prepare the Sensual Space with your partner, lighting candles, lighting incense, collecting pillows, and playing soothing background music.** Make sure both of you are being responsible in preparing and cleaning up your shared space.

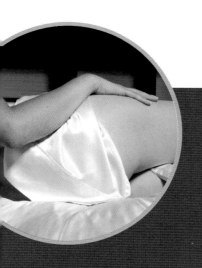

"I'm amazed at how **releasing negativity can change an evening.** Tonight I was so mad at my partner I didn't think I could do the date night as planned. I consented at least to the Opening

Sit opposite each other, and set the timer for your two-minute Weather Reports. Have you made Coming Clean a regular ritual, or do you have withholds that keep you occupied in judgments and fear? What can you offer to clear the air? What needs to be said that has not been said? If you haven't Come Clean in several days, do it now.

3. **Clear away negative energy.** What are you feeling in this moment that will not serve a juicy, rich night of sensual sharing and exploration? Get rid of it. Name it, and with your partner's help, swish it away together with hand gestures. Be gone—out the window or door! Now you both become like religious caretakers who sanctify your space and make it abundant with luscious attributes such as love, sweetness, beauty, truth, and respect. Ask that passion, honor, and joy rain down from the sky so you may be awash in them. Call them in with arms opened to the heavens, and feel graciousness trickle down upon you.

4. **State your intentions as the "Master and Mistress of Will" that you are.** What do you claim, decree, and create for tonight? Intend it and see how magic happens. Energy follows thought. What do you intend for your night of discovery? "I intend to be a magical child." Stretch yourself with statements such as, "I intend to fall deeper in love with life" or, "I intend to have a pleasure orgasm" or, "I intend to solve the mystery of the universe." If you don't intend it, it will not happen, and if you do intend it—it could happen!

5. **Come into the body by setting the timer for three minutes of Soul Gazing and Ocean Breathing with your partner.** Make your breath bigger than ever before. Profound breathing is the root core of erotic sex. Push your envelope. Because we are given only a finite number of breaths for our lifetime (somber, but true), decide to maximize each one. Shallow breathing, like when you're sitting at the computer, gives you a computer experience; deep and slow breathing, best when you're having sex, gives you a profound experience.

Ritual and offered to release my anger toward him. It really worked! Instead of postponing our date night and feeling self-righteous—and lonely all night—I moved on to a great and loving evening. **The Opening Ritual is powerful."**

—LESLIE, AGE 38

6. **After coming into the body, the partner with the darkest hair sets the timer for two minutes and asks the other, "What do you appreciate about me?"** The other speaks for the whole time, sincerely, voicing the little and big things he or she loves about you. At the end of two minutes, breathe in all the glory and say, "Thank you." Often, we let compliments slide off our back or even belittle ourselves with remarks like, "Well, I used to do it better," or, "So-and-so does it better," or, "Yes, but you didn't see the time I screwed up," etc. We often disperse our discomfort in "receiving" by quickly returning a compliment. Don't do it. Let self-doubt fly out the window now (if you haven't already released it in your negative clearing).

7. **After two minutes of telling your partner what you appreciate, present your gift to him or her.** The listening partner should receive the gift as a small token of his or her inherent worth and experience. Open it, and give thanks. Reset the timer, and trade roles.

Erotic Exercise 2: Blindfolded Ceremony of Sensual Delights   [SEVENTY MINUTES]

In this exercise, you will blindfold your partner for thirty minutes and nonverbally offer him or her sensual tastes, sounds, smells, and touch to awaken his or her body senses. In this fun and sexy exercise you get to tease, play with, and stimulate your partner in all kinds of ways. You become the master Magician of Pleasure, orchestrating a sensual feast on his or her body. You become the Trickster of Tease and entrap him or her in your web of surprise and suspense, whetting his or her appetite for more.

Taking It In

Accepting compliments, like good sex, takes practice: Practice taking it in when someone compliments you. Let a compliment soak into your very core. Breathe it into your bones. Allow it to settle and feel cherished. It's that simple. Own your experience. Own your skills, talents, and knowledge; by standing tall, you extend a quiet hand and pull others up to your level. Good sex and compliments are about surrender; by taking in, we graciously give back.

Now it's time to prepare for the Ceremony of Sensual Delights. Decide who will give first (the woman, in this example). Spend five minutes preparing a plate of your taste and sensory treats in the kitchen. Cut into small bite sizes several fruits, vegetables, cheeses, and sweets, and have several liquids available, like water, wine, and liquors in small glasses. This exercise is not about eating; a small taste can be savored more easily than big bites that require a lot of chewing.

Think of textures while selecting food, such as what may feel smooth and melting on the tongue and what may be surprisingly thick or crunchy. Think of cool and warm, moist and dry. Get a variety, probably at least a dozen food samples plus several liquids. Collect sensory tools such as feathers, furs, and essential oil misters. Perhaps you have prepared ahead and bought a surprise touch toy from a sex shop. Also prepare sound treats for the ears, such as finger cymbals, a Tibetan bowl, or bells and a chime. Include several essential oils on your sensual palette for opening the most primitive sense of all, olfactory. Wash your hands when finished with your preparations.

While the woman is preparing the food treats and sensory props, the man prepares for the ceremony by arranging himself on a throne of pillows from which to be pleasured. Perhaps you'll don a special silk robe. Sit back on your throne, blindfold yourself, and breathe the Sexual Breath you learned during the last Erotic Night. Breathe in for five counts (five seconds, or adjust to your liking), hold the breath in at the top for another five counts, then exhale slowly for five counts, and hold the breath out for another five. Have you been practicing your PC Pulses? Add them to the slow, four-part sexual breath. Prepare your body for the Ceremony of Sensual Delights just as you would any sexual encounter—with breathing that is deep and slow.

Sex and Tease

Most women say they don't get enough teasing and lament that men are wired to go right for the goods. In my years as a sex coach, I've been surprised how often I hear men lament, "She just wants to do it one way and rather quickly at that." We've lost the art of slowness, tease, and play in sexuality. Containing sexual energy without letting it spill over into overt sexual touch or penetration is a lost art in our hurried lives. Often we don't take the time to design a sensual feast; orchestrate intrigue; or move toward, then away from the target in sex. Tease is an art form worth refining for any lover.

When ready, the woman brings in the taste treats for the Ceremony of Sensual Delights and checks that her partner's blindfold is secure and comfortable. Tell your man that, for the next thirty minutes (set the timer), he is to lay back, take in, and enjoy the delights you have prepared for him. You will not be talking, so that both of you can stay in a body (rather than a head) space. Instruct your man to ask for anything he needs, such as covering up for warmth or adjusting pillows.

Breathe into his ear your slow, hot, moist breath. Remind him you will be taking care of him. He may lose his mind and come to his senses wandering directionless into erotic realms. If he slips into a shallow breath, guide him into a profound experience by coaxing him into deeper breath. Model for him slow, Sexual Breathing. Just hearing your breath will reassure him of your connection.

Start with opening an essential oil and quietly placing it under his nose without touching him. Let him drink in the scent. If he talks, remind that him sounds are fine, but not words. Lightly tingle a bell at one ear. Pause, then move it to the other ear. Stroke his ears with a feather. Work silently so he does not know what to expect. Come toward his body with gentle moves that are smooth, secure, and safe feeling—yet full of surprise and discovery. Spray scented mist several feet above his head, and let it drift over his face and limbs. Space your treats; do not rush.

Try using both hands at the same time—stroke his hair while feathering his inner thighs. Two senses at once are good. Use your full hand and forearms in order to contact more skin with your touch. Choose another scent to put under his nose to awaken the primordial brain. Lightly chime a Tibetan bowl directly over his head, and as the sound ripples out, move the bowl toward one ear, then the other. Loosely let your hair fall over his chest and face. Use your lips and tongue to softly tease and suck on his nipples, then blow a stream of cool air on them.

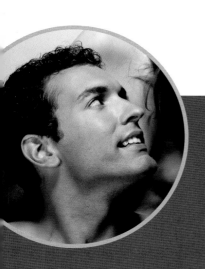

"When she whispered in my ear, 'Stay with your breath, your sensations, and your pleasure. **This is about you; I want you to surrender to your senses and abandon your**

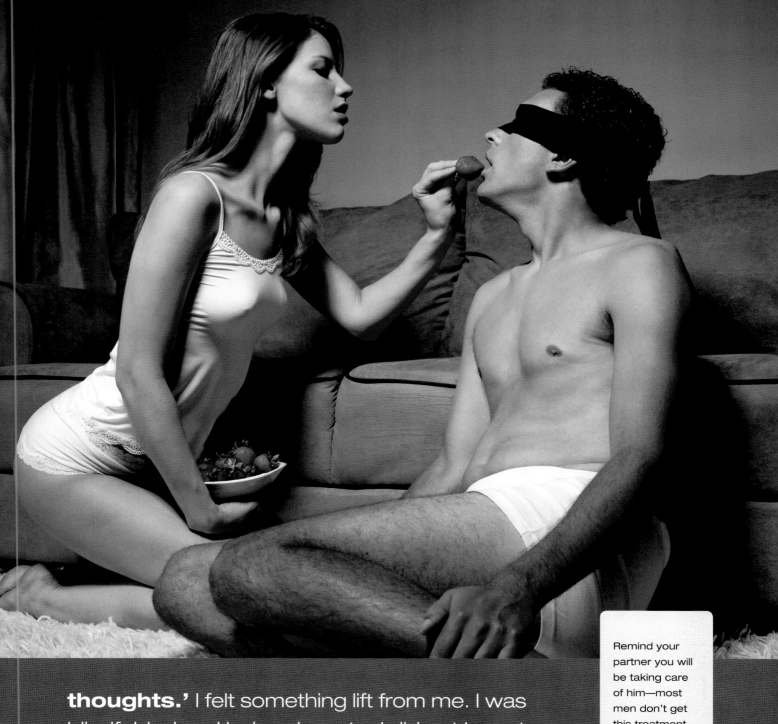

thoughts.' I felt something lift from me. I was blindfolded and being done-to. I did not have to be in control. **Surrender was my only job, and I loved it."**

—BRUCE, AGE 37

Remind your partner you will be taking care of him—most men don't get this treatment enough.

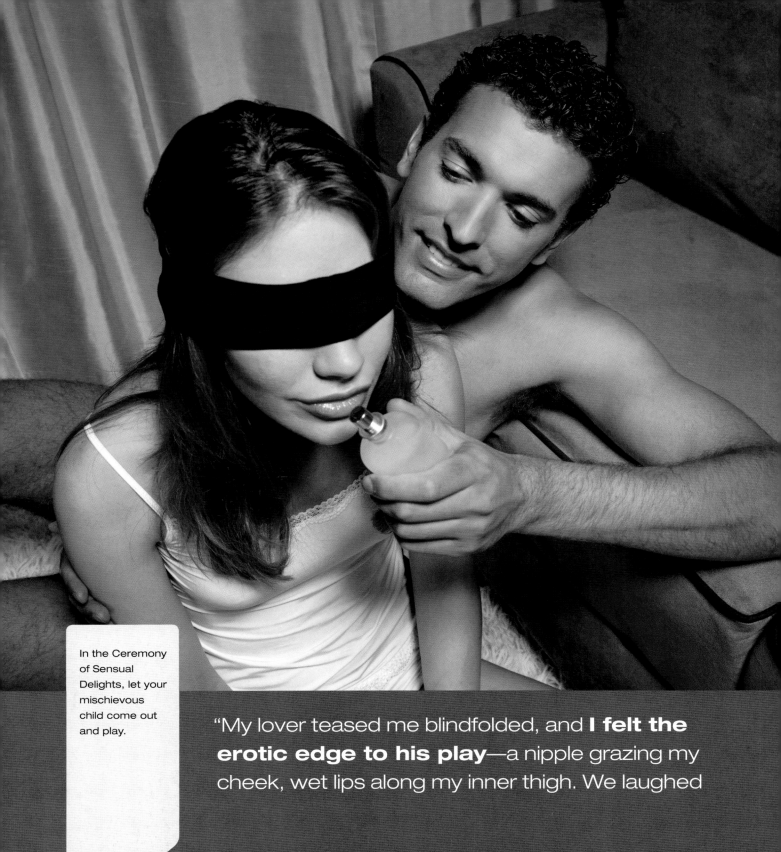

In the Ceremony of Sensual Delights, let your mischievous child come out and play.

"My lover teased me blindfolded, and **I felt the erotic edge to his play**—a nipple grazing my cheek, wet lips along my inner thigh. We laughed

Begin your blind taste treats. Choose a light food like a cucumber or melon slice, and brush it lightly over his lips. Repeat with a firmer stroke, wetting the lips and even dripping some juice on his chin. Slip the juicy morsel into his mouth—and take it out again teasingly. Play with the slippery melon over his tongue and teeth, and then finally let him eat it. Watch him savor the taste. Pause thirty seconds or so between bites; being leisurely gives him time to enjoy the mysterious texture and flavors. No talking.

Stay with a light food for the first three or four tastings. Use your fingers provocatively in and around his mouth. Lick away any drips from the corners of his mouth. Give him a sip of water to clean his palette. To really tease him, purposely let some water spill as you give him a sip. Giggle and lovingly, playfully wipe him off with a soft cloth.

We're being naughty here, doing everything Mother told us not to do with food. Go for some stronger tastes like avocado or a strawberry. Allow him to smell it first. Brush the texture across his lips. Squish it gently against his teeth. Pause and watch him discover the flavor. Try some cheese. Put a wine goblet up to his mouth, and let him sip. Taste the wine on his lips lightly with your tongue. Feed him a crunchy cracker for surprise.

Consciously design your taste treats. For example, give him a peeled grape in between two cheeses. Use sherbet (or water) to cleanse the palette after a strong taste. Toward the end, bring out the sweets and liqueur. Do not rush. Tasting should take about twenty minutes or so. Invent the play as you go, breaking the rules, inviting your mischievous child to take charge.

At the end of thirty minutes, take the leftover plate of morsels out of sight, slowly take off his blindfold, and do a Heart Salutation. Refrain from talking about what you fed him or did to him. Stay nonverbal and in a body space while exchanging roles. The man goes to the kitchen to quickly prepare his food treats and collect his sensory props (in five minutes, while the woman prepares her throne and blindfold to receive. She breathes the five-count Sexual Breath in preparation.

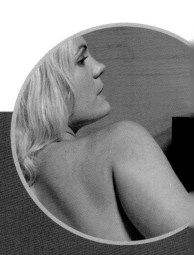

for no reason, especially after a surprise taste of lemon! We aren't usually this frivolous; **our sex will be flavored by this treat."**

—GEORGEANNE, AGE 41

Erotic Exercise 3: Self-Pleasuring
with Your Partner as Witness   [EIGHTY MINUTES]

In this exercise you have the opportunity to take the most common of all sexual acts, masturbation, and shed the silence and shame surrounding it by touching yourself and your genitals in front of your partner. By sharing this usually hidden act, you expose your solo-sexuality to another, inviting expansiveness, and surprising heat. It's hot to see your partner turned on, and you can learn subtle things about his arousal.

When asked "Who was your first lover?" you probably think of your first intercourse experience. But actually, you were probably your own first lover, and you may have begun as a teenager or earlier. Masturbation, or Self-Pleasuring, is the most common, most performed, and most natural of all sexual acts. Yet it is veiled in shame, silence, and guilt. You probably felt pressured to hide it, thinking you were wrong or dirty to touch yourself, and feeling you were the only one who did it.

Hence, you developed self-touch techniques that are fast, repetitious, and quiet—you didn't want to get caught, and you can't be creative when you can't talk about it! These traits become the mainstay of solo sex, yet they are not traits for good partner sex. Your genitals become the most touched part of the body, but with the least creativity. Habitually, you use the same strokes, positions, time, and place to Self-Pleasure as you have for years—or decades. Old conditioning founded in shame still runs the program. Tonight you are about to change that for a real, juicy jolt to your sex life.

Seeing your partner in the vulnerable state of self-arousal is hot, hot, hot! You feel relieved that you don't have to do anything or be responsible for his turn-on. Who gives whom an orgasm, anyway? Witnessing your partner take charge of his pleasure becomes hotter when you don't feel the pressure to perform.

When I had to do this exercise in my sexology training, I thought I would die. I figured someone was really going to be bored (and me embarrassed) for how lackluster my self-touch habits were. But by the end of the hour, I was amazed at where I went, what I did, and how this exercise opened me to greater sexual enjoyment.

If you think this exercise may be too difficult to do, look at it this way. You would probably love to have a lover luxuriate over your body for thirty-five minutes (or more). So be that lover. Rub lotion on your body, feather your face, tickle your inner thighs, caress your genitals, and touch for you, for fun, for pleasure, without design, without outcome. Spend timeless and treasured moments exploring your own body erotic, and someone will want a piece of that action.

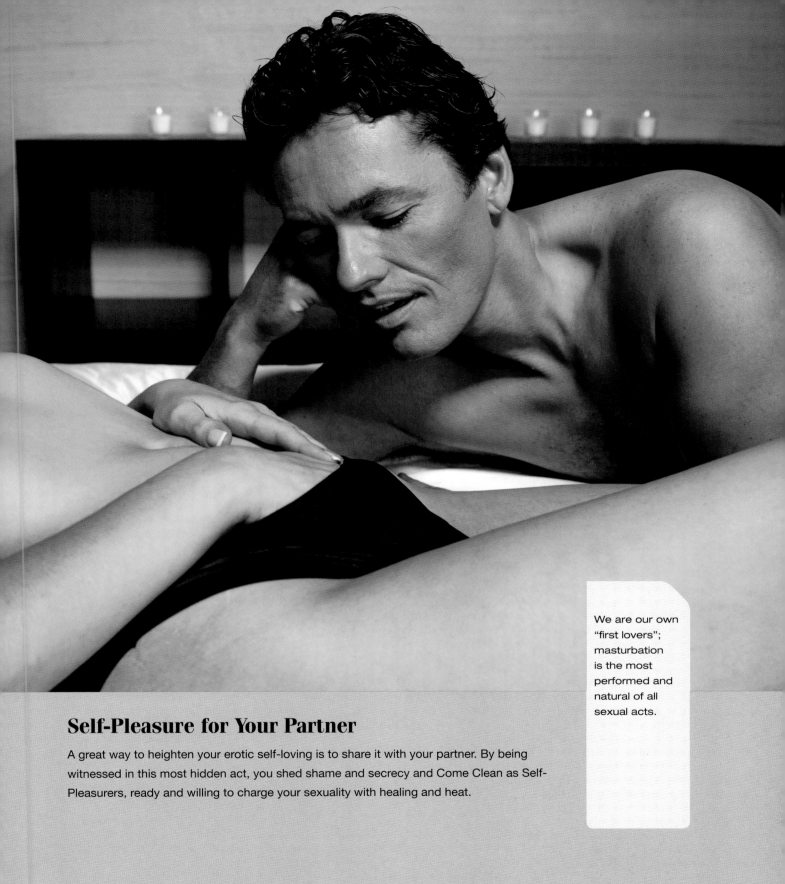

We are our own "first lovers"; masturbation is the most performed and natural of all sexual acts.

Self-Pleasure for Your Partner

A great way to heighten your erotic self-loving is to share it with your partner. By being witnessed in this most hidden act, you shed shame and secrecy and Come Clean as Self-Pleasurers, ready and willing to charge your sexuality with healing and heat.

WOMAN SELF-PLEASURING

Decide who will go first (the woman in this case), and arrange any props, lubricant, and lotions, you would like for your Self-Pleasuring session. Sit opposite your man, and Soul Gaze and Ocean Breathe together. Take a minute to set an intention for your session, such as, "I intend to play lovingly with myself," or, "I intend to be a sassy, sexy wench." As a witness, the man also sets an intention, such as, "I intend to support to my partner lovingly" or, "I intend to appreciate my partner's exploration." The witness sits comfortably where he can see but not interfere with the Self-Pleasuring partner.

Set the timer for thirty-five minutes, and play music you enjoy. Start by closing your eyes (wear a blindfold if you'd like) and centering attention onto yourself either standing or sitting on your throne. Be conscious of your breathing. If it is shallow, listen for the ocean sound coming in and out. Though you are being witnessed, this is for you; bring your attention to your body, and say to yourself several times "for me."

Sway, dance, or meditate to the music until you notice a desire to touch yourself in some way. Do not feel rushed to go to the genitals. Sense your whole body as a fine instrument with which to play. Let your intuition lead your hands over your body, caressing your neck and collar bone, teasing yourself. Do you feel like misting your face . . . smelling some scented massage oil . . . licking the rim with your tongue . . . feathering your lips or pussy . . . rubbing scented oil on your nipples, or licking if off a shoulder?

When your mind wanders to the thought of being watched, bring your attention back to the sensations you feel from touching your own skin. Touch yourself for your pleasure, for your sensations, and without needing to go anywhere. This is an internal experience for you.

Touch your genitals with curiosity and interest. The clitoris does not lubricate, so rub a little oil on the magic button. Play with the petals of your lotus flower, dip into the hot, holy well—the Source of All Life—and spread the nectar in circular motions around the sensitive vaginal opening. With a finger and more lube, reach inside about an inch to the wrinkly, spongy goddess-spot of the vaginal wall behind the pubic bone.

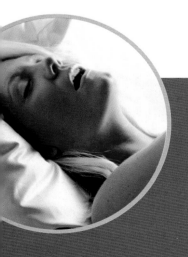

"I couldn't believe **how much more sexy I felt being watched** than being alone. Before I would never masturbate unless my husband was out of town—ha! Here he was in the same room.

Massage this gorgeous erectile tissue that is internally connected to the clitoris. Women wear their erections on the inside. Explore in all directions this interior moist cave of mysteries. Feel the knob cervix at the end. Feel the outside opening of the urethra getting plush and soft with stimulation. Do not pressure yourself to get wet or have an orgasm, although it is fine if you do. Enjoy your exploration for each moment. If you find yourself holding your breath, stop and breathe until you relax into the moment again.

When the timer sounds, wash your hands and sit opposite your partner. Set the timer for two minutes, and tell what it was like for you to be witnessed Self-Pleasuring. Set the timer for two more minutes so your partner can tell you what his experience as witness was like. It's not a time to judge techniques but rather express in positive terms your own experience. End in a Heart Salutation.

MAN SELF-PLEASURING

Sitting opposite one another, the man takes a minute to state his intention for Self-Pleasuring, and the woman states her intention for witnessing. The man sets the timer for thirty-five minutes, plays music of his choosing, and has lubricant handy. The woman sits comfortably where she can see and not interfere.

Either standing or sitting on the throne, wearing a blindfold if desired, begin the internal process of connecting with your body and intention through a deep, slow breath. Close your eyes, connect with your breath, go into your body, and tune into your desires. Though you are being witnessed, this is for you. Keep bringing your attention back to your body and your sensations. Feel your whole body as a sensual playground. Move around, looking at yourself in the mirror if you'd like.

Feel your strength, your power, and your ability to protect and provide. Feel your jaw, whiskers, and Adam's apple. Most women are fascinated by these male traits. Touch or massage your strong arms and shoulders, perhaps with lotion. Rub oil on your solid, manly hands. Believe me, she is watching every move. Put oil on your chest. Pinch and play with your nipples.

I've missed playing with myself since I've been married, and now **I've reclaimed the joy of Self-Pleasuring** . . . and my husband is my biggest fan."

—JEANNINE, AGE 43

For fun, feather your inner thighs, feet, genitals, and ass. Put lotion on your legs and thighs, the most powerful parts of the body. Lovingly admire your strength and willingness to serve others, and let the lotion as well as your self-gratitude soak into your body. Massage your butt cheeks just how you like it. She's probably squirming and taking note.

Play with your balls dry before any putting on lubricant. Grip the skin between your fingers, stretch it around, and massage it between your fingers. This skin's sensitivity is analogous to the inner lips and vagina on a woman. Play with your cock without lube; stretch it long and wiggle it. Be playful. Let go of needing to be or get erect; just enjoy all states of this fascinating appendage—she does!

Liberally put massage oil or lotion on your balls and cock. Stroke up from your perineum area (the pelvic floor behind the balls and in front of the anus). This is called "the hidden cock" and feels wonderful. Most women do not know that almost half of your cock is behind your balls, and it feels great to massage and play in this area. By enjoying yourself, you show her what you like.

Put lots of lube on your cock, and try stroking with new techniques, rhythms, pressures, and speeds. Mix it up. Play with the shaft as well as the head; alternate between the two. Massage your heart area while you massage your cock. Enjoy your unique cock, its veins, mushroom head (for stroking the g-spot), and deep rosy color. Perhaps externally massage the sensitive anus. This under-appreciated and over-shamed part of the body plays a big role in enhancing male potency and pleasure. The anus is a major erogenous zone for both men and women, and for a man it's the gateway to your internal g-spot, or prostate gland. Internal prostate massage brings waves of bliss and multiple orgasmic ripples throughout the entire body.

Do not feel like you need to ejaculate. It's fine if it happens and also fine if you contain your sexual potency. You have a choice. You always have a choice. You may choose a few seconds of explosive genital orgasm or choose to remain in extended periods of whole body orgasmic realms. When the timer sounds, wash your hands, and come back to sitting in front of your partner. Set the timer for two minutes, and share with your partner what the experience was like for you. Then give her two minutes to tell her experience as witness. End in a Heart Salutation.

Erotic Exercise 4: Closing Ritual   [TEN MINUTES]

Tonight you have honored the body erotic by giving each other a sensual feast and sharing your solo ritual of masturbation in front of your partner. Be gentle with one another in this vulnerable state.

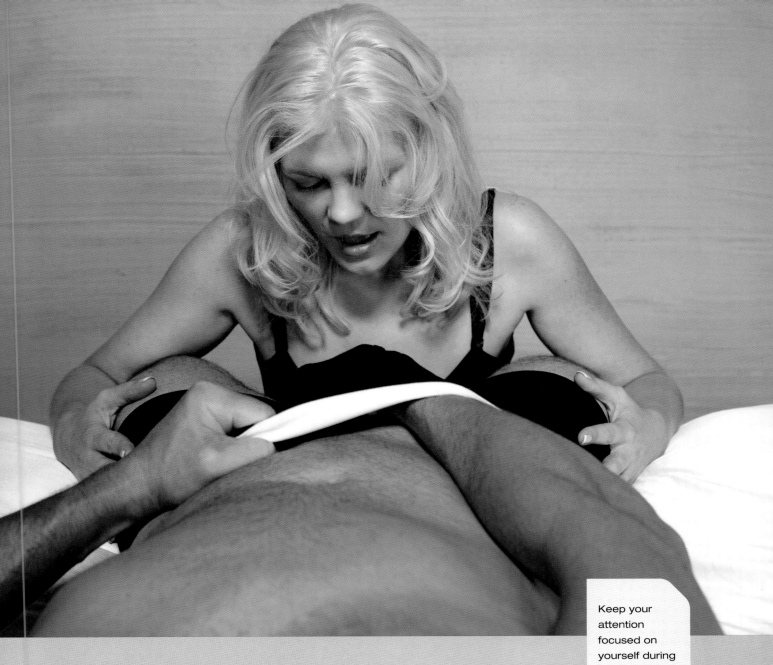

Respect Your Penis

Approach your cock with an attitude of respect. Instead of being a little critter hooked to the front of you that is never doing the right thing, make whatever your cock is doing the right thing, and adjust your attitude to fit it. This wise and wonderful part of you loves play without being coerced to be one way or the other. As you play, enjoy subtle stages of arousal without pressure to go anywhere. Most women love playing with penises in all stages of hard and softness.

Keep your attention focused on yourself during Self-Pleasuring. Though you are being witnessed, this is for you.

Revisit your agreements on confidentiality and containment, or refraining from sexual intercourse, this evening. Perform your closing gesture, clean the Sensual Space, blow out candles, and leave the space before resuming normal conversation.

Looking Ahead

Read Erotic Night Six. I suggest dividing up this next night (on Healing Genital Massage) into two 2-hour evenings instead of one 3-hour night. That way neither partner has to give an erotic massage just after receiving one. In addition, you will have added time to bathe your partner before the massage, which can be very euphoric. Decide now with your partner whether to stay with the original schedule or add a second night (both scenarios will be discussed). If you choose to spread the Erotic Night over two nights, have a bath pillow, bubble bath, and bath oils and salts on hand for each.

Try Self-Pleasuring at the same time with one another for a hot night's adventure. Shower together and then set the timer for forty minutes and simultaneously Self-Pleasure.

Erotic Recap

- Opening Ritual: *twenty minutes*
- Blindfolded Ceremony of Sensual Delights: *seventy minutes*
- Self-Pleasuring with Your Partner as Witness: *eighty minutes*
- Closing Ritual: *ten minutes*

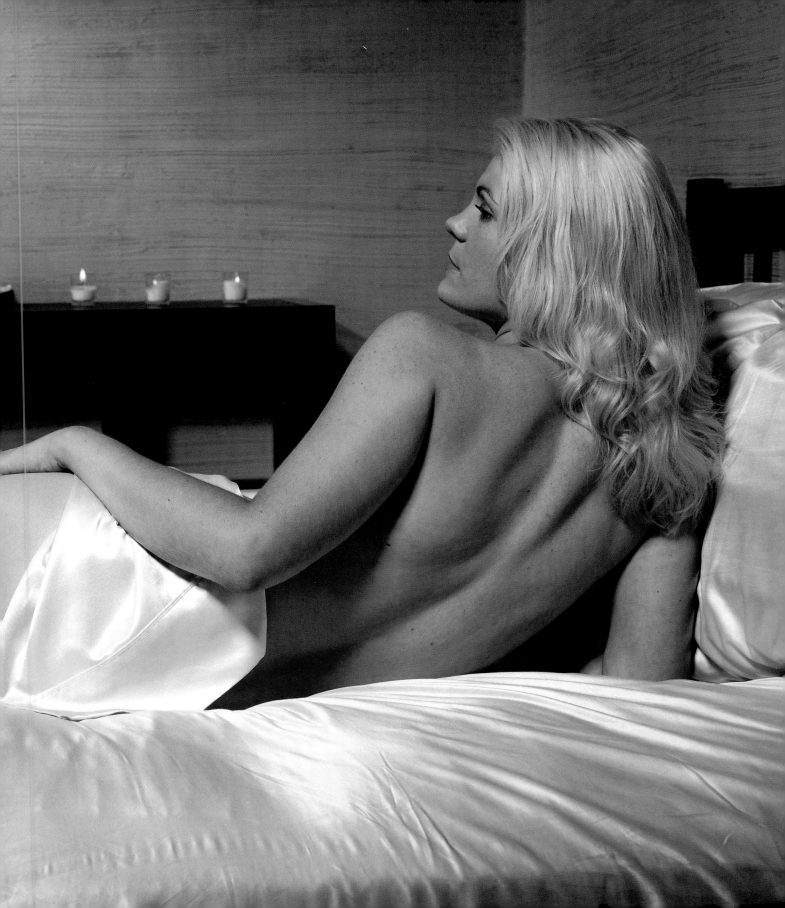

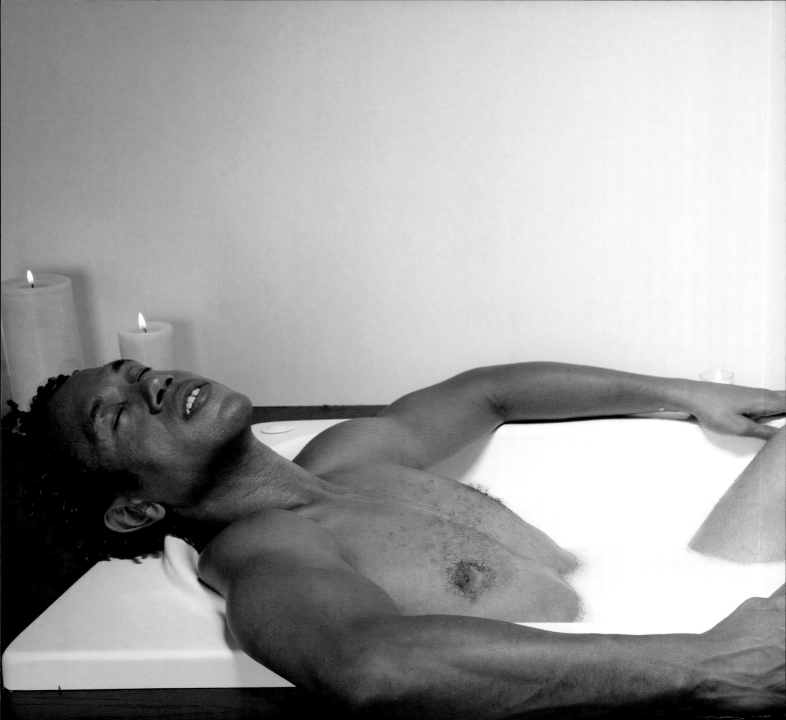

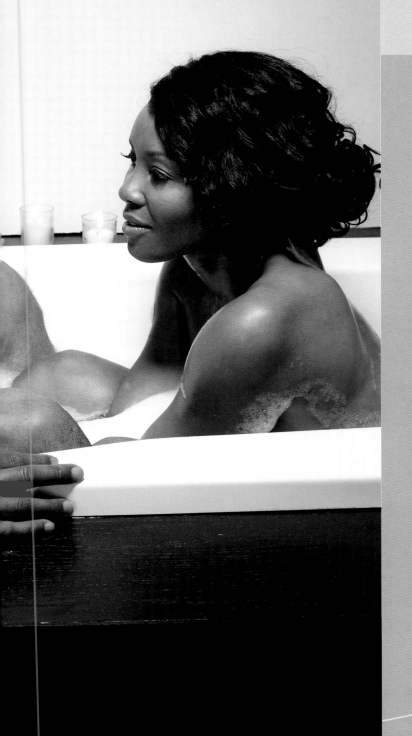

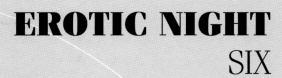

Healing Your
Partner with
Erotic Genital
Massage

EROTIC NIGHT
SIX

During the previous Erotic Night, you gave your partner a Blindfolded Ceremony of Sensual Delights and Self-Pleasured for each other in the spirit of honoring your body temple and sharing self-eroticism. Tonight you will massage your partner's genitals to restore and revitalize his or her erotic potential.

You are a powerful healer for your partner, and stepping up to this sacred role is yet another way you can empower your sexual relationship. All of us have difficult issues around sexuality. Perhaps you have felt pressured into sex when all you wanted was to cuddle, or you have started down the path to intercourse and changed your mind but could not express yourself. Perhaps an older person made you feel uncomfortable or abused you when you were too young to do something about it.

Your tissues store these negative memories, which can numb and chronically tense your pelvic region, blocking your sexual organs from pleasurable sensations. Massaging your partner's genitals with the intent to heal past sexual disappointments and shame invites greater sexual ease, joy, and grace back into lovemaking. Giving your partner a Healing Genital Massage melts and softens the body's armor and resistance around the genitals and opens the pelvis to greater movement and freedom for your best loving yet.

If you have elected to put aside two nights for this exercise, follow the outline below. If you have chosen to do both partners in one night, skip the Sensual Bath, and add ten minutes each to the Body Caress and Genital Massage portions of the evening.

Make preparations for the Sensual Bath. About twenty minutes before the start of the Opening Ritual, the giver cleans and fills the tub with hot, bubbly water and adds fine bath salts and essential oils (perhaps lavender) and maybe some fresh rose petals. Have on-hand a large bath towel, two hand towels, fine soap, and a salt or sugar body scrub. Light the room with candles, and keep it warm and steamy. If convenient, have soft music ready to play. Also have your massage bed (or table) prepared for after the bath with clean sheets, lube, a hand towel, pillows for under the knees, and a blanket.

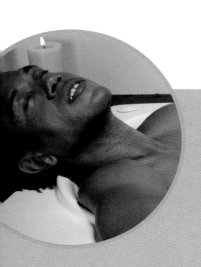

The Love Pump

The Love Pump (Kegel or PC muscle) pulses the rich, hot, root energy from the genitals up through the body's inner flute, or spinal column, to warm the heart and open the body's center of intuition located between the eyes, referred to as the Third Eye in Tantra. Every cell in the body is saturated, sensitized, and invigorated by the rising heat from the fiery, red root. Your genitals are the body's furnace, and the Love Pump circulates the fire to heat the whole "building."

Erotic Exercise 1: **Opening Ritual** [FIFTEEN MINUTES]

Both partners, groomed and dressed in bathrobes, show up on time for the Opening Ritual, ready to be present with one another, willing to tell the truth, and ready to open your hearts to any outcome the powerful evening may take.

1. **Prepare your Sensual Space with music and candles.**

2. **Sit on pillows on the floor facing one another** cross-legged with knees touching or with the woman's legs loosely over the man's thighs.

3. **Set the timer for each of your two-minute Weather Reports and Come Cleans.** Clear the sacred air for the deep sharing to come. Cleanse your Sensual Space by releasing negative fears and doubts about the evening and calling upon positive energy to surround your ceremony.

4. **Set your Intention for the Healing Genital Massage,** such as, "I intend to heal my partner with touch and attention tonight" if you are the giver or, "I intend to open my genitals to love and healing" if you are the receiver.

THE TANTRIC KISS

Set the timer for five minutes for a Tantric Kiss with Sexual Breathing and PC Pulses. The woman sits yab-yum position on the man's lap. Gaze and breathe several sounding breaths together. Come into a loose kiss, and synchronize your breathing, slowing it down and putting in a pause after the inhale and exhale. You do not have to silently count, just aim at a mutually agreeable slow pattern, with pauses at top and bottom, and stay together.

When the rhythm feels comfortable, the man changes into alternate breathing so he exhales when the woman is inhaling. Keep the pauses together. Bring awareness to your body sensations, merging, dissolving, and vibrating with the pleasure of your own breathing. Come into wonder. Surrender into the love inherent in every moment. Pulse your Love Pump during any pauses you desire; for variety, try a fast flutter or long squeezes with holds. After weeks of daily exercising, you probably feel the power of a stronger pelvic floor muscle and know why it's called the love muscle. End in a Heart Salutation.

Erotic Exercise 2: **Sensual Bath Ceremony**   [THIRTY MINUTES EACH]

The giver (in this case, the man) leads the woman into the bathroom and sets the timer for thirty minutes. Have her check the water temperature and adjust it if needed; the hotter the better, as long as it is comfortable. Gently disrobe your woman, and assist her into the tub. Use a bath pillow or a hand towel to support her neck and head. Kneeling beside the tub, drape a soaked hand towel over her abdomen and breasts for added warmth. Let her know you will not be talking much in this honoring and purifying ritual so you both can enjoy a body space.

1. **Encourage her to lie back and feel her sensations.** Softly sighing with each exhale, connect in your breathing, and place your hands over her heart. She may choose to close her eyes. Start by slowly rubbing a sugar or salt scrub onto her upper chest, shoulders, and neck. Rinse her off by wringing the hand towel onto her body, and then resoak the towel in tub water and slowly pull it up over her genitals and breasts for added warmth.

2. **Support her arm in your arm, and massage the scrub gently into her limb all the way out through her hands and fingertips.** Check with her about the pressure and speed of your strokes. One never complains of a massage being too slow. Every few minutes, resoak the hand towel in hot tub water, and pull it back over her chest for added warmth. Continue slowly with the other arm and hand.

3. **Massage the feet with liberal amounts of body scrub.** Feet are connected internally to the sex organs; suck her toes if you desire. Remember to refresh the soaked towel with hot water and recover her breasts. Work up the body one leg and thigh at a time.

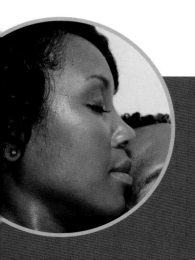

"For as long as we have been together, this is the first bath my partner has given me, actually **the first 'being bathed' that I ever remember.** I felt like I was a baby being bathed by a nurturing caretaker, and I totally surrendered.

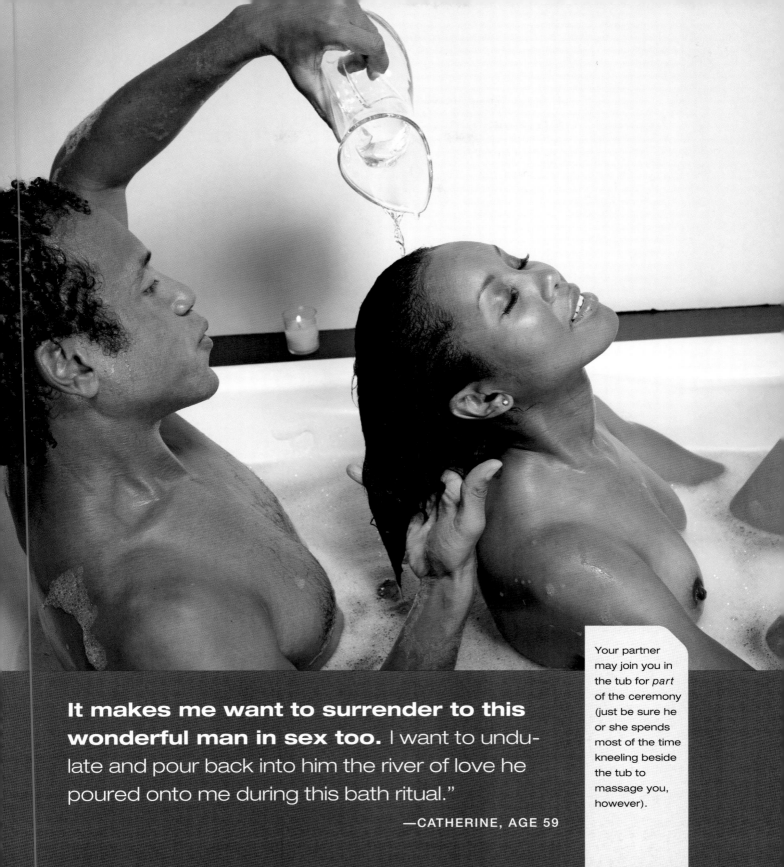

It makes me want to surrender to this wonderful man in sex too. I want to undulate and pour back into him the river of love he poured onto me during this bath ritual."

—CATHERINE, AGE 59

Your partner may join you in the tub for *part* of the ceremony (just be sure he or she spends most of the time kneeling beside the tub to massage you, however).

4. **Pace yourself so you may caress the whole body in the given time frame without rushing.** You are orchestrating the experience—keep an eye on the timer so you may seamlessly transition and cover each part. Slip a soapy hand, not the scrub, over the genitals, resting your palm on her pubic bone.

5. **Massage her inner thighs where they meet the torso with the other hand.** Do not directly finger the genitals or go inside her vagina; rather, use your whole hand to cup and vibrate the genital region. Pet her pussy with a slippery hand-over-hand stroke from between her legs up over the pubic mound.

6. **Continue with soap up the abdomen and breasts.** Have her lean forward and scrub her back with the textured scrub. Her back body is tougher than her front body, so you can use more pressure. Rinse the back with the hand towel.

7. **With a few minutes to go, help her step out of the tub slowly, and begin drying her body with gentle pats and slow strokes.** She may lean against a wall for the back body. Lead her silently onto the bed, floor pad, or massage table for a Body Caress and Healing Genital Massage.

Erotic Exercise 3: Body Caressing [THIRTY MINUTES EACH]

Honoring the whole body is important before giving a Healing Genital Massage; cherish the whole body before touching the most precious, vulnerable parts. Assume the role of reverent caretaker, and pour your sacred attention into this healing ceremony. Adjust the music, set the timer for thirty minutes, and have her lie on her stomach.

Pay special attention to teasing the genitals from the back body. Stroke up the inner thighs. Massage the crease where the thighs meet the torso. Feel deep for the sit bones and make massage circles around them. These movements indirectly tease and stimulate the clitoris. Jiggle the fleshy butt cheeks. If she tenses, tell her to relax her buns like jelly.

After about fifteen minutes, ask her to turn over for a frontal caress. She may feel cooler with her stomach exposed. Ask her if she'd like a silk scarf or blanket draped over her abdomen. Cool bodies tense up, impeding surrender, whereas heat encourages letting go and openness. Remind her to follow her breath and her sensations, because she will feel more vulnerable touched on this sensitive side of the body. Breathe with audible sighs to encourage her relaxation.

Use some of the front caress techniques you have reviewed from Erotic Night Three, including the heart/genital hold. Ask her for permission to touch her breasts. Casually pass over the genitals on your long, slow body stroking without singling them out. Don't forget the bottoms of the feet. If she's ticklish, try slightly more pressure and ask her to stay connected to the touch. Don't give up; the feet are sex organs too.

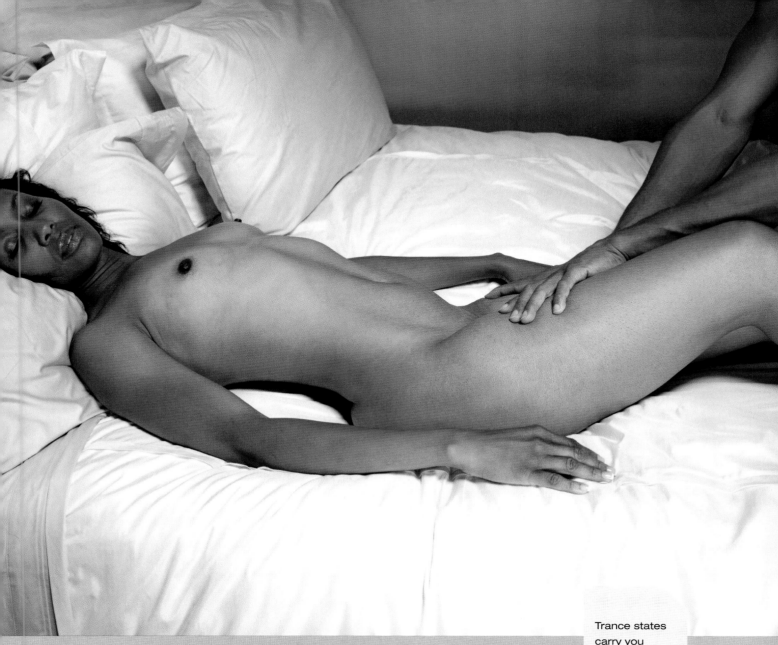

Entering a Trance State

Allow yourself as a giver to float into a trance state. It will encourage her to do the same.
Receiving is the hardest role; it's the position of less control and most uncertainty. As giver,
model surrender for her by letting go of your own expectations and floating into the timeless
realm of whole body wonder and awe.

Trance states
carry you
beyond the
particular and
into the divine.

Erotic Exercise 4: **Female Healing Genital Massage** [THIRTY-FIVE MINUTES]

Ask for permission to touch her genitals, and speak aloud again your intention for doing so. Set the timer for thirty-five minutes. Remind her that this is not about preparing her for partner sex or penetration. The power of this massage comes from a one-way gesture of respect and gratitude without the expectation or orientation of sex. You are touching to encourage healing and release past disrespect and harm done to her. Let her know that if emotional things come up, you will support her in feeling her feelings, without judging or trying to fix anything.

As you touch the genitals, be aware that the negative experiences stored in the tissues may come out in unpredictable, emotional ways. Commit to being there for your partner with whatever comes up in the moment. Tell her you have no expectations beyond being there to support her. Remind her that she does not have to get wet or orgasm, but it's okay if that happens. Your intention is to help heal past fear and anger in order to inspire a new level of truth, trust, and loving in your sexuality.

EXPLORE THE AREA (FIVE MINUTES)

Positioned at her heart, or left side, place your hand over her heart and the other palm over her pubic bone with cupped fingers covering her genitals. Soul Gaze and breathe together. Establish connection before moving. Gently start vibrating the genital hand (and arm) as a whole unit. Keeping one hand on her heart, trace a path with the genital hand over the abdomen to her heart and back several times.

Exhale slowly a deep sigh of hot air about an inch away from her *yoni*, or vulva. Spread the outer vulva lips apart with both hands, and sigh more hot sighs onto the newly exposed pink petals. Breathe in deeply, and blow a stream of cool air onto this region. Cover her lower abdomen with one hand, and with the other, trace a U-shape from the inside of one knee, up the thigh, over the genitals, and down to the other knee. Repeat this stroke several times.

Take a large pinch of her labia, or outer vulva lips, between your thumb and first finger. Pull, shake, vibrate, and massage it firmly between your fingers. Do not be timid. Ask her about pressure. Continue this stroke every half-inch or so down to the vaginal opening and then up the other side. Massage firmly the perineum between the anus and vagina, but do not enter the vagina. Be mindful not to touch the anus. While it is a wonderfully erotic zone (and subject for another massage), unless you can assure her you know the proper hygiene protocol, she'll worry about getting a vaginal infection and not be present to your touch. Play instead with her pubic hair. With a palm securely resting on the pubic bone, press down and make deep circles, indirectly manipulating the clitoris.

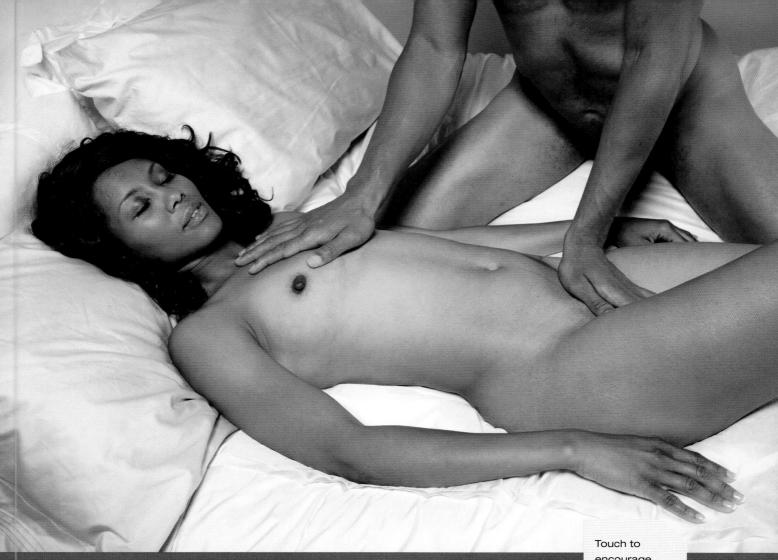

"Entering a healing place with genital touch was new for me. I felt awkward at first that I was not giving back, but then **I felt surprisingly relaxed and even excited** that this was not going to end in intercourse. I realize how breaking old routines heightens attention and love for my partner."

—MARIA, AGE 37

Touch to encourage healing and release the past disrespect and harm that was done to her.

PLAY WITH THE MAGIC BUTTON (FIVE MINUTES)

Put a generous amount of lubricant on your fingers, and lightly pet her genital area hand over hand. With slippery fingers, make soft circles around the clitoris, and ask her, "Would you like more or less pressure?" Also circle around the vaginal opening. Vary this stroke with different rhythms, pressures, and vibrations. Include pauses while touching the clitoris; this area, like the head of your penis, needs pauses in stimulation. Go slowly. Be aware that neither of you hold your breath but, rather, engage in deep, slow Ocean Breathing.

Slide your fingers slowly up and down the valleys on each side of the hooded clitoris and vaginal opening. Vibrate this stroke, and change it in slight ways. Tap lightly on the clitoral hood; does she want it stronger, faster? Be creative. Remember her Self-Pleasuring strokes, and mimic them. Try pulling the hood of the clitoris back to expose the shiny, lentil-size glans, and then release it, sliding it back and forth repeatedly. Ask her, "How can I make this experience better for you?"

ENTER THE TEMPLE GATES (TEN MINUTES)

Ask most reverently for permission to go inside, saying something like, "May I enter your garden of pleasure?" or, "May I come inside your deepest being?" or, "May I put a finger inside of you?" With permission, put more lube on your fingers and massage around the vaginal opening without rushing in. Enter her "holy well" as a priest would enter heaven's gates.

Once inside the hot, moist "purse of pleasure," hold still. Energetically, this is a big shift. Generally men tend to be doers and move too much. Feel your ability to penetrate her internal experiences silently, absorbing and releasing what needs to pass without moving. Begin exploring tenderly; can you can feel how some of the areas are smoother and denser than others inside this cave of mysteries?

Close to the vaginal entrance and under the pubic bone, feel the egg-shaped, spongy tissue hanging down from the top of the vagina. This sensitive g-spot area on the top side of the vagina has two deep valleys on each side and goes back a full finger's length. It has ridges and feels wrinkly. Called the female prostate, when stimulated, this area on the roof of the vagina engorges just like a penis. Ask her if she feels a particularly sensitive area of her vagina, and give it loving attention.

On the g-spot, curve your fingers toward the pubic bone as if to motion someone to come to you; stroke her in a "come to me" gesture. Pause and repeat several times. Feel the "gutters" that run down both sides of the g-spot, defining it. Feel the sensitive "tail" of the g-spot all the way in about a finger's length. What kind of pressure does she like on it?

Try pressing up firmly on the g-spot toward the pubic bone, holding, and then vibrating for a few seconds. Release and breathe; try this several more times, with pauses in between. Move your fingers in a back-and-forth motion like a windshield wiper over the

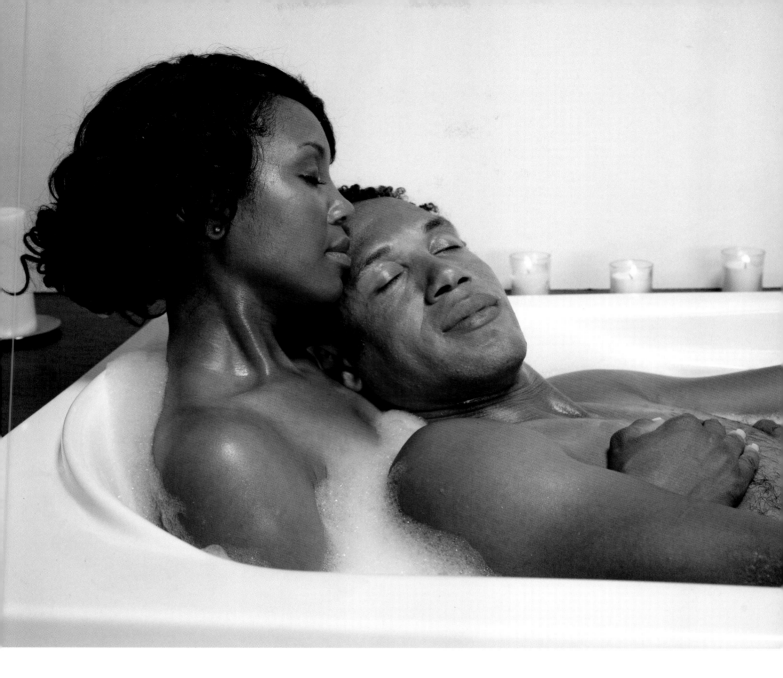

g-spot. Start with lighter pressure, then move more energetically and consider giving very vigorous strokes. Remember to use your skills of asking whether she would like it slower, faster, harder, lighter, longer, or shorter.

A Healing Genital Massage is a time to use communication skills. Instead of worrying that talking will ruin a sexual experience, this sacred time is dedicated to healing. Encourage her to talk and even to name what she is ready to let go of. If she prefers silence, know healing comes in many forms.

MASSAGE INTERNALLY AND EXTERNALLY (TEN MINUTES)

Keeping your finger(s) inside, move the hand resting on her abdomen so you can manipulate the hood of the clitoris between your thumb and first finger. Alternate stimulating the clitoris with internal g-spot work, ten seconds on one, then the other, and then pause. Less is more. Often, just when a woman loves something her moans encourage the man to go faster and deeper, when actually being consistent and steady is what she wants. Let her come to you; be solid in your presence, and she can bear down more against you when she desires.

It's easy, when getting to the genitals, to forget to focus on your own sensations and get caught up in the performance of pleasing another. If you remain with your intention of allowing her to release, you will find your meditative center in this ritual.

COME TO STILLNESS (FIVE MINUTES)

With five minutes left in the massage, tell her you are going to come out of her. Come out slowly, as you would leave a holy temple. Cup your moist, warm hand over the external vaginal opening, and leave it there for a minute or so, alternating between holding still and

You become a powerful healer for your partner by giving a Healing Genital Massage.

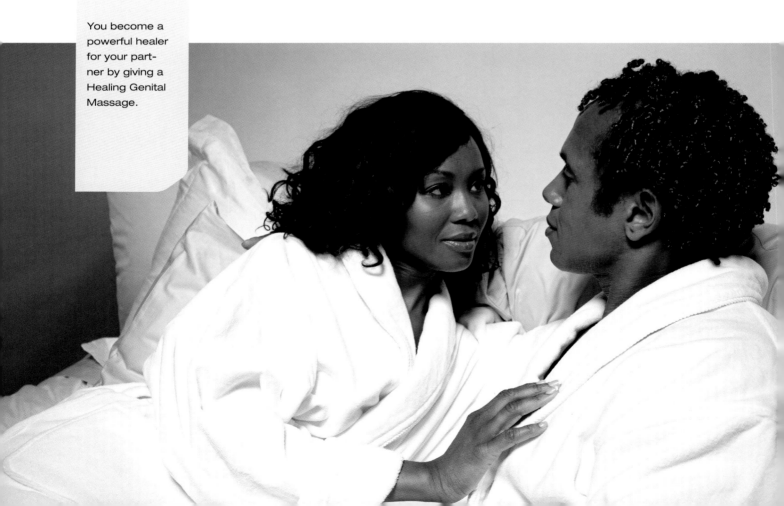

making small vibrations. With your other hand, gently massage the abdomen over the womb in slow circles.

Keeping one hand on the genitals, lightly stroke with the other hand up around her shoulders and neck and down the arms. Switch hands on the *yoni* and in long, sweeping strokes, float a hand over the legs to the feet and back several times. These connecting strokes integrate the genitals to the body and act as finishing strokes for the massage. End with your hands back on the heart and genitals for a few breaths together. Healing often comes in layers; don't expect everything to change with one ritual. Commit to revisiting this modality for healing again and again.

Cover her with a robe or blanket, and tell her to remain there as long as she wants and that you'll return for the closing ritual in awhile. Leave the room. With genital touch, you may think the only right ending is intercourse and orgasm, so you may feel strange leaving her. However, you are expanding your repertoire of approaches to sexuality and the body. Absorbing the experience is best done individually. Come back into the room after a few minutes, help her on with her robe, share a Heart Salutation, and do the Closing Ritual.

Erotic Exercise 5: Male Healing Genital Massage   [THIRTY-FIVE MINUTES]

You may worry if your penis isn't erect (all the time) that your partner might not think you are turned on and enjoying her touch. Or you may be so concerned about the angle of your penis (erect or not) that you often miss the enjoyment of feeling subtle sensations of arousal in your body. And if you are preoccupied with being responsible for your partner's happiness, you may be holding back or pushing ahead to please her rather than going at the pace that is right for you. Men need to "not do"—that is why this massage is so healing for you.

Soft or Hard

The penis doesn't have to be hard for a great experience. Tell your man that you enjoy touching his penis whether it's soft, medium, or hard. The hardness of his penis, just like the amount you get wet, is usually independent of your loving feeling for him. Tell him that you love playing with him in all stages—soft-on to hard-on. Let him know his self-worth is independent of the angle of his penis.

EXPLORE THE AREA (FIVE MINUTES)

Remind your man there is no agenda, achievement, or "right" outcome for this massage except for him to take it in and enjoy all his sensations without concern of being hard or soft. He doesn't have to get hard, stay hard, or ejaculate, though it's okay if he does. The receiving role is particularly difficult for a man, but in receiving, he learns how to give to you and how to surrender into ecstasy. Begin the exercise much like the Female Genital Massage. Begin Soul Gazing, Ocean Breathing, connecting the heart and genitals, and U-strokes along the inner thighs.

Take scrotum skin, analogous to the inner lips of the vulva, between your thumb and index finger, and roll it around. Try this in different places over the scrotum. Take the head of his penis in your hand, and pull up on it, gently shaking it. Play with his pubic hair, chest, and nipples.

MASSAGE THE MAGIC WAND (TWENTY MINUTES)

In Tantra the penis is called the Jade Stalk or Wand of Light. It is a creator of new souls. With an attitude of reverence, lay your hand with fingers spread out over the penis, and pour massage oil over both. With one hand on the heart and the other on the genitals, begin gently and slowly massaging and vibrating with both hands.

Create strokes that are light and playful on the penis, not those designed to get him hard or aroused. Stroke in a way that is not his habitual way to make love or masturbate. This will allow his penis to get resensitized to a greater variety of feeling. Enjoy what you can do with a soft penis. Stretch it "around the clock," massaging it in all directions. Don't be hurried; touch for you. If you're trying to get him hard, you're working too hard and need to drop back. Remember to breathe deeply and slowly, and it will guide your touching.

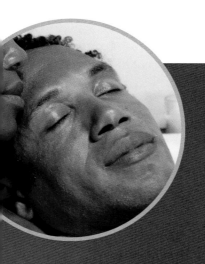

"The last time I was touched like this, I was a baby. Of course, I don't remember it exactly, but I feel that is how I was **nurtured, loved, and cherished** as an infant. **This massage was incredible;** I went back to my very beginning."

—STEPHEN, AGE 47

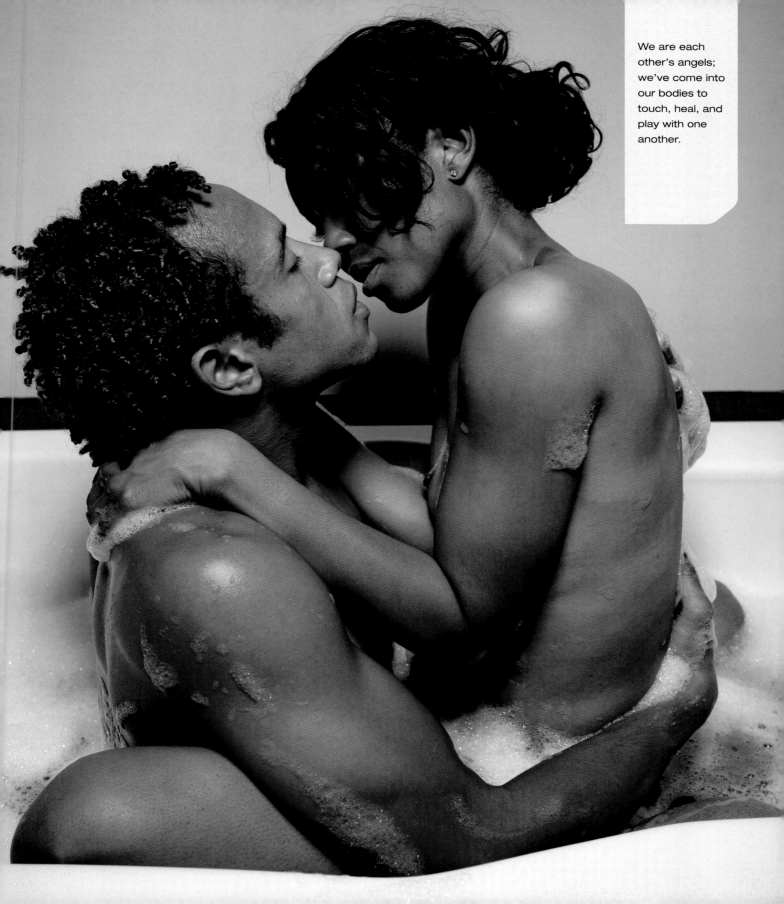

We are each
other's angels;
we've come into
our bodies to
touch, heal, and
play with one
another.

Try holding the base or shaft with one hand, pulling the sensitive skin around the head more taunt, and playing with the head, or glans, with the other hand. Lightly stimulate the head as if you were juicing an orange. For another stroke, use a corkscrew motion, holding the base of the penis with one hand and twisting up from the bottom to the head and back down again with the other hand. Check with him about pressure and speed. Vary strokes with pauses and vibrations for interest. Remembering his strokes from the Self-Pleasuring exercise, and mimic and play with variations on them here.

Use the whole penis in your touching. Include strokes on the shaft, a less sensitive area, to give the sensitive head a rest from arousal. With one hand stroking the penis, use the other hand to stroke his inner thighs, abdomen, and chest, thus dispersing erotic energy throughout the body. Alternate strokes on the penis with strokes on the perineum.

MASSAGE THE PERINEUM, THE HIDDEN PENIS (FIVE MINUTES)

Almost half of a man's penis is behind the balls and in front of the anus. This Hidden Penis is rarely discovered by women, but it's much appreciated when it is. When this root perineum area is massaged, the genital fire is spread out over a larger area, helping a man to prolong his erection and arousal. Make a fist, place it on the perineum, and firmly press up toward the heart, using all your body weight. Rotate your fist to massage his sit bones. Hold and vibrate. This area needs a lot of pressure. Open your hand, and cup it over the perineum, massaging and pressing firmly, and place your other hand over his heart. Massage the space where the legs meet the torso of the body. Let a feeling of acceptance flow from you to him however his penis is.

CONNECT THE GENITALS TO THE WHOLE BODY (FIVE MINUTES)

This section is the same as for the woman. Refer back to the "Coming to Stillness" section for ending the Healing Genital Massage.

Erotic Exercise 6: Closing Ritual   [FIVE MINUTES]

Tonight you gave or received (and perhaps both) a Body Caress and Healing Genital Massage. Bask in the relaxed joy of prolonged and heightened rapport you've gained with your partner from these gifts. Feel in your body, whether you gave or received, how a Healing Genital Massage opens the hert to greater loving.

Repeat your Closing Ritual gesture and/or saying. Blow out the candles and leave the space. Refresh your agreements of confidentiality and containment of sexual energy for the rest of the evening. The giver cleans up the massage and bath space. The receiver may take time to jot down feelings in his or her Ecstasy Journal or simply rest. You may ask each other for permission to visit the happenings in Sensual Space later and share your experiences.

Looking Ahead

- Read Erotic Night Seven before it takes place.

- Make a Yang List (see page 145) and give it to your partner five days ahead of the next Erotic Night. Keep another copy of your list in your Ecstasy Journal for you.

- Prepare for any items that you choose from your partner's Yang List comfortably in advance of the next evening date.

Erotic Recap

- Opening Ritual: *fifteen minutes*
- Sensual Bath Ceremony: *thirty minutes each*
- Body Caressing: *thirty minutes each*
- Female Healing Genital Massage: *thirty-five minutes*
- Male Healing Genital Massage: *thirty-five minutes*
- Closing Ritual: *five minutes*

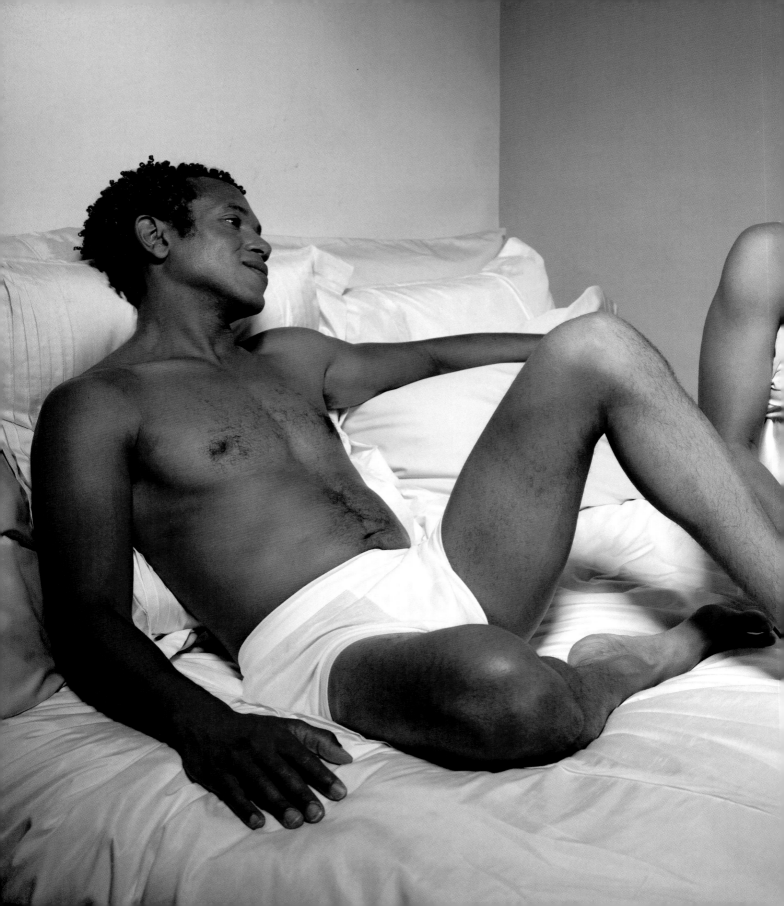

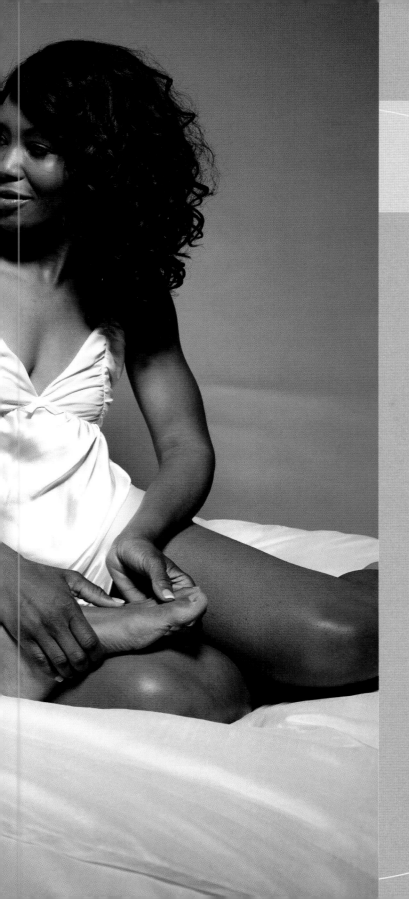

EROTIC NIGHT
SEVEN

Playing with
Power and
Surrender
in Intimacy

EROTIC NIGHT
SEVEN

During the previous Erotic Night(s), you gave your partner a Sensual Bath, Body Caress, and Healing Genital Massage, and you also received the same gifts. Tonight the man will invite his "inner female" and the woman her "inner man" out to play for a frolic into spicy, sexual turn-on. You will dip into the deep well of power and surrender dynamics, both to enrich your personal growth and excite relationship play.

You want to be powerful in the world. You want all your wishes to be fulfilled, for others to serve you, and to utterly control the outcome. You aspire to be Master of the Universe. And on the other hand, you long to give it up, to let someone else be in charge, to utterly surrender, and to not have to initiate the next move. Just as traits of exhibitionist and voyeur are part of your nature, so are the tendencies to enjoy having power over as well as submitting to another.

An intimate relationship is the perfect place to discover, learn from, and play with the dynamics of power and surrender in a safe, sane, and consensual environment. The Erotic Nights you have experienced so far have been designed to build truth and trust in your relationship so that you feel safe enough to step out of the small box of the "right" way to have sex and step into the larger arena of fearless loving with more risk-taking, edges, and surprises.

Infidelity in relationships can result from boredom caused by lack of discovery, fun, and play between couples. Couples get stuck in inflexible roles and feel insecure about stepping outside of the box. Feeling uncreative at home, you think a new face, a new sexual position, or a new intrigue will solve your boredom, when actually you need to challenge your limits by going deeper into the love of a truthful and trusted relationship. Playing in a conscious and safe way with power and surrender deepens relationship love by bringing freshness, aliveness, and unpredictability to tantalize you. You're a kid at heart. When did you stop playing at sex? When can you start again? Playing the Yin/Yang Game tonight will fuel-inject excitement in your lifetime of great sex.

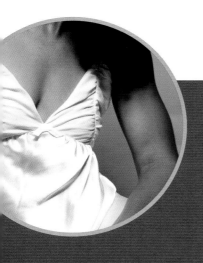

"Before I used to think that **being dominant or submissive** with a partner meant your relationship was unhealthy and you needed dark and scary things to feel excited. After playing the

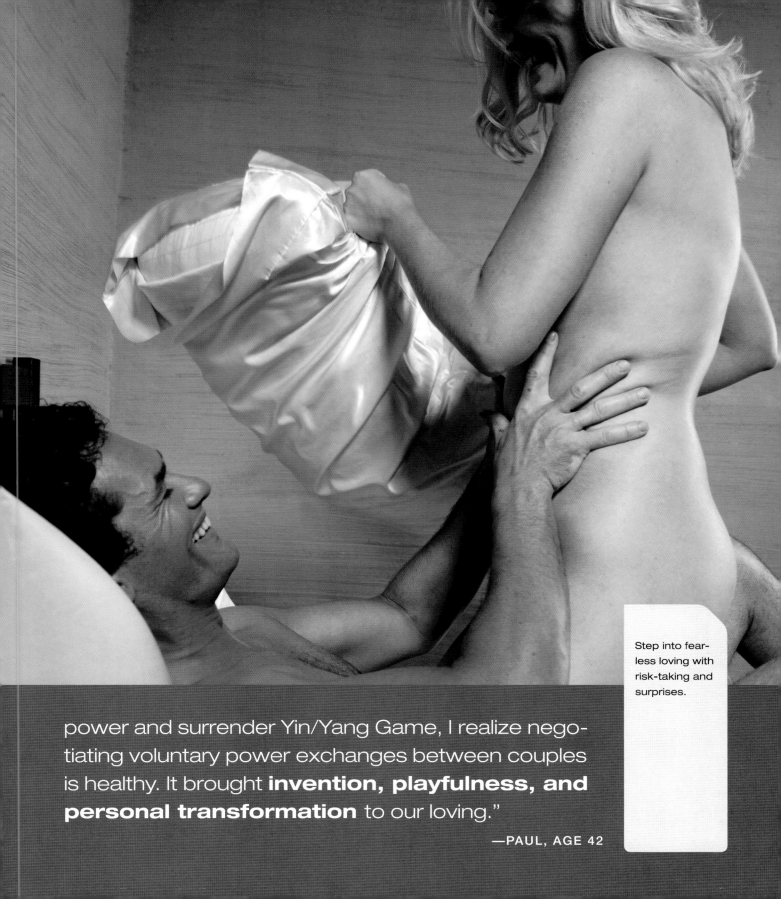

Step into fear-
less loving with
risk-taking and
surprises.

power and surrender Yin/Yang Game, I realize negotiating voluntary power exchanges between couples
is healthy. It brought **invention, playfulness, and
personal transformation** to our loving."

—PAUL, AGE 42

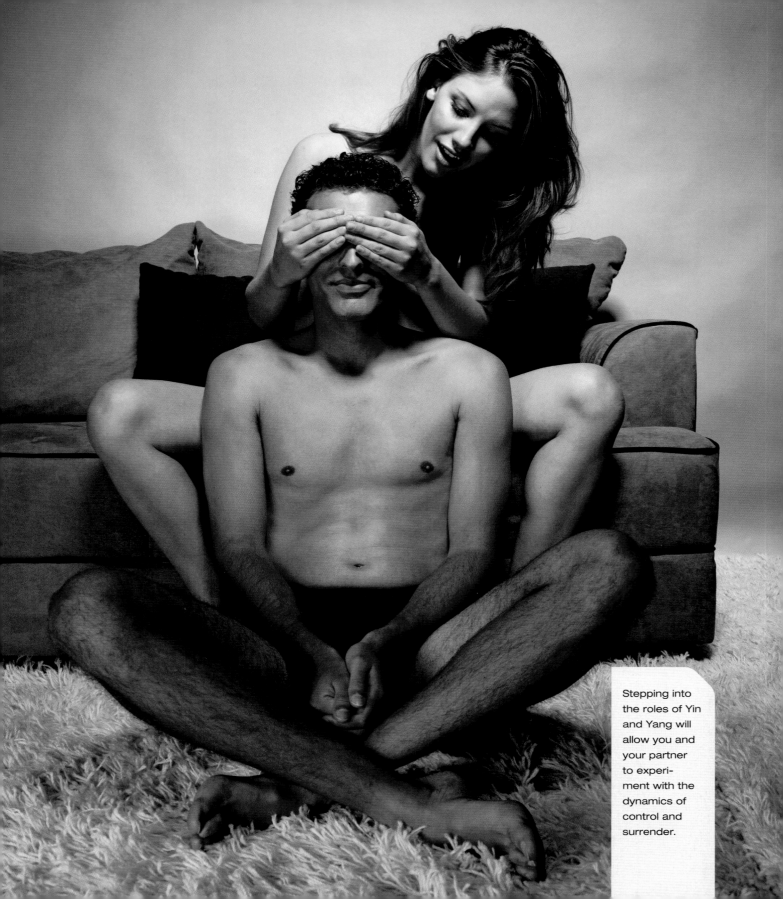

Stepping into the roles of Yin and Yang will allow you and your partner to experiment with the dynamics of control and surrender.

Preparing for the Yin/Yang Game

Yang in the Eastern tradition represents the male principle of being active, in control, or dominant; Yin is the female principle of being receptive, submitting, or surrendering. Eastern religions seek a balance between the opposing yet complementary principles of Yin/Yang that is missing in our Western cosmology, in which images of the divine are primarily male. Even though Western stories of origin lack a divine balance, you don't have to be stuck in one way, such as always doing (Yang) or always being done to (Yin). You can seek balance in your personal life and relationships for joy and expansion.

To play the Yin/Yang Game, one of you makes wishes (Yang), and the other fulfills those wishes (Yin). Separating the roles helps you learn to make wishes and enjoy making others' wishes come true. You may feel inhibited about asking for what you want and feel being "wishful" is wrong. This game will exercise your Yang muscle of taking command, directing the erotic show, and being in charge. You will also have a turn at Yin, where you put "me" aside and surrender "your way" in order to serve and nurture the other. If you've ever said no to another's request in order to stay in control, you'll see that being Yin expands your view of pleasure and excitement through the lens of your partner's sexuality.

The Erotic Night is divided in half, so each partner will get to experience a balance of initiating and yielding. In real life, a flow between these two polarities is healthy and enlivening. Often one partner feels stronger in one role, say the woman in being Yin and the man in being Yang, so playing both roles offers an opportunity to look at yourselves and expand the balance and flow of give-and-take in a relationship—and outside of it. Similar to the Three-Minute Game you have already played in this book, the Yin/Yang Game expands the opportunities and dynamics of leading and following.

MAKE YOUR YANG LIST

To begin, you need to make a Yang List of everything you want your partner to give or do for you. Your partner, of course, will also be making up a Yang List. Just making the list will get your fantasy juices running and add zest and zaniness to your erotic imagination.

To make your Yang List, write down in your Ecstasy Journal everything you as "Master Designer of Your Ecstasy" may like your Yin servant to perform, gift, or do for you. At first there are no limits of time or money; at this point do not think about what your servant may be willing to give or how to fit it into one evening. Unbridled in your enthusiasm to be pleasured—Queen (or King) of the Universe that you are!—make believe, as if by a stroke of the pen, anything is possible. This is not a time to be shy or have self-doubts. Ladies and Gentlemen, start your engines. Here are a few examples to get your creative juices going:

- Serve me (naked except for a bow tie) breakfast in bed for two, with fruit crepes, real maple syrup, a poem, and flower blossoms.

- Lead me blindfolded through the park, teasing me with touch textures and taste treats from the natural environment.

- Pose naked for me in sexy photographs or videos.

- Dress up in sexy clothes, dance a strip-tease, and lap dance for me.

- Brush my hair and stroke my face, and caress my front, back, and genitals.

- Give me a foot bath, massage and kiss my feet, suck my toes, and put nail polish on my toes while you sing praises to my beauty.

- Hold me like a baby for an hour, rocking and stroking, and tell me you love me.

- Gift me with flowers, a new shirt, fancy underpants, jewelry, lingerie, chocolate, etc., and include with the gift an original poem about your love for me.

- Tell me an original, sexy bedtime story, and tuck me into bed stoking my hair.

- Read me aloud a hot, steamy erotic story that turns you on, too. Look up at me between the lines.

- Lay on top of me naked for thirty minutes of meditative Body Bonding (see page 43).

- Let me dress you up in my clothes, and you role-play me flirting and asking you out for our first date as if we had just met.

- Seduce me on the kitchen table or counter or floor or. . .

- Tie me up naked (without leaving me unattended and agreeing upon a safe word that tells you to untie me at any time), and tease me with feathers, furs, and tickling. (If bondage play is new to you, read *SM 101* by Jay Wiseman first.)

- Spank me (check with me for pressure first) and tell me what a naughty child I am for doing all those bad things to the neighbor boy, and then give me luscious aftercare. (Safe word stops the play.)

- Tell me how many ways you love me and all the things you want to do to me.

- After a Sensual Bath, give me a full-body massage for an hour and a half.

Have fun making your detailed Yang List. After you've finished your exhaustive and comprehensive list of ways your partner can please you, read it over. Obviously there's no way you could get all that goodness and pleasure packed into one night. That is why this game is most effectively played over a larger time frame, such as a whole evening, or better yet, a whole weekend—for twenty-four hours you are Yang, and for the next twenty-four hours you are Yin.

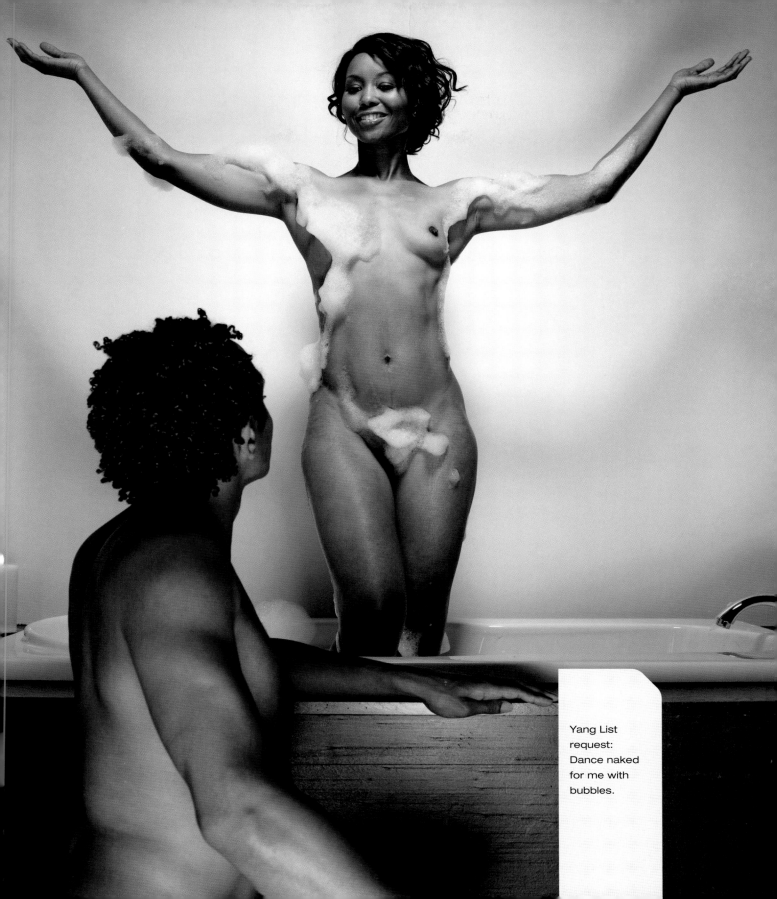

Yang List
request:
Dance naked
for me with
bubbles.

PRIORITIZING YOUR YANG LIST FOR YOUR PARTNER

Going back over your Yang List, decide what you desire most for your pleasure in a block of time lasting seventy-five minutes, or about one-half of the power and surrender evening. Review the list with your particular Yin servant in mind; what may he or she particularly relish in serving you?

With your partner's erotic palette in mind, underline and prioritize with numbers the activities on your Yang List that you most want for your Yang time. Suggest time frames for each of the activities. For example, you may underline "Dress up in sexy clothes, dance a strip-tease . . .," add a priority number and time frame, and jot any additional instructions for your partner. Go on down your list, selecting, underlining, and adding time frames and any notes. The following are activities selected, prioritized, and timed from the sample Yang List that would add up to seventy-five minutes:

1. Dress up in sexy clothes, dance (you can pick the outfit and the music, two songs at about three minutes each): ten minutes

2. Gift me with flowers and jewelry (I'd like an original poem about your love for me that rhymes and is child-like): ten minutes

3. Read me aloud a hot, steamy erotic story that turns you on (feel free to touch yourself while you are reading and looking up at me): ten minutes

4. Spank me (pull my pants down and put me over your knee), tell me the naughty things I did with the neighbor boy, and then pat and lightly stroke my bottom with love: ten minutes

5. Hold me and rock me like a baby (I may suck my thumb): ten minutes

6. Give me a foot bath, massage my feet with love, and nibble my toes: twenty-five minutes

Make a copy of your list with priorities underlined, numbered, and timed. Then exchange your complete Yang Lists (not just your priorities) with your partner at least five days in advance of the next evening date. It's helpful to see not only your selections but also the

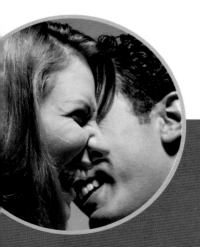

"Receiving my partner's Yang List was like **looking through a window into his sensual soul. I** loved seeing all the ways he wanted me to cherish

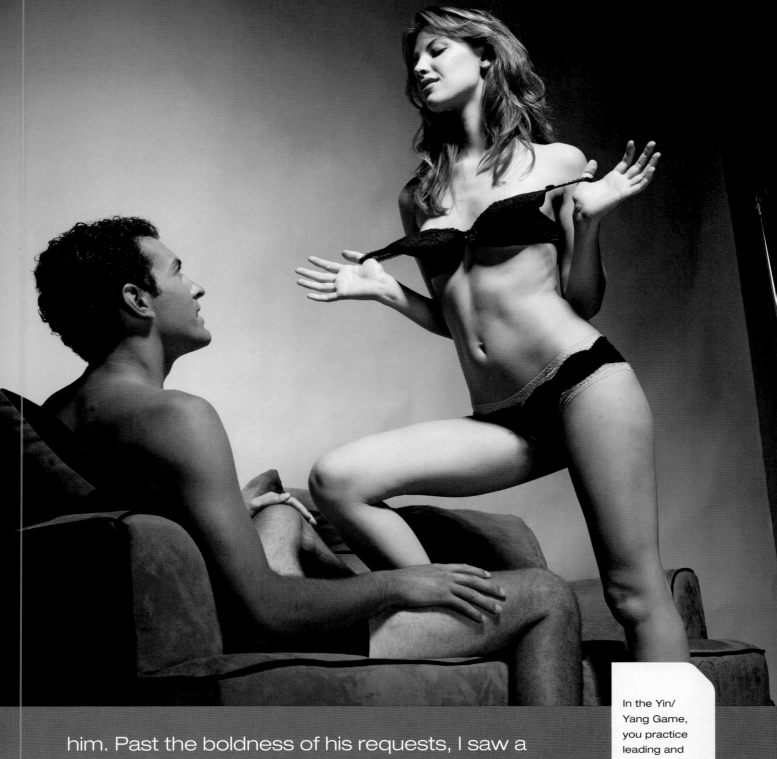

him. Past the boldness of his requests, I saw a vulnerable little boy tugging at his Mother's apron strings wanting more love. And I get to serve him!"

—BRENDA, AGE 46

In the Yin/Yang Game, you practice leading and following by taking turns initiating play and yielding to your partner.

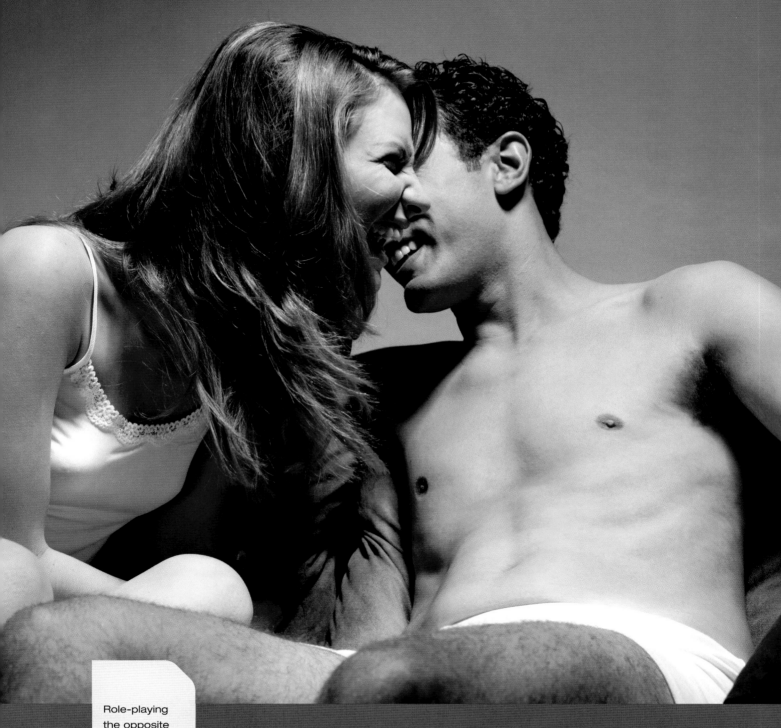

Role-playing the opposite gender is fun—and revealing. You'll see yourself with new eyes.

"I couldn't believe **how funny it was** to see him acting as me. I didn't even realize I did the things he was acting out. For me to move and speak and take on his manly traits felt like trying whole spectrum of your wishes. You are not tied to this list on the night of play; it is a start. You may wish—and are free to—make changes during actual play.

As Yin partner, receive your partner's Yang List, and prepare to serve your partner according to his wishes as long as it pleases you, too. Kindly substitute any of the activities you prefer not to do with ones you will enjoy submitting to. You may ask for help, "I'm not comfortable selecting erotica at the bookstore; could you bring home a book from which I can choose a story to read you?" Do your shopping and preparations well in advance so you arrive on time, groomed, rested, and ready to play on the date night.

Erotic Exercise 1: Opening Ritual: Role-Playing Your Partner   [FIFTEEN MINUTES]

In the spirit of playful discovery, you are going to role-play your partner during the fifteen minute Opening Ritual. Dress in his robe or attire, and walk into the room assuming his gait, stance, body movements, and mannerisms. You do not often get to see yourself through another's eyes. You can touch your own masculinity or femininity in new ways by role-playing the opposite gender. In this mutual exchange of roles, you can see more clearly the fixed attitudes you carry about being a man or a woman.

You'll find yourself laughing, but at the same time seeing deep revelations in your merriment and parody. For the whole ritual, including Weather Reports, Come Cleans, Creating Sensual Space, and Body Caresses, submerge yourself in the other's personality, the way he talks, what he talks about, how he gestures, and how he listens and carries his body. Take on his name for the ritual, act like you worked his job, and share as if you lived his day.

Playact every aspect of his behavior. Exaggerate a bit to make your observations clearer. Though much will be humorous, be disciplined in your new roles so that the game can work. Even if you feel you can't mimic all the details of your partner, stay with the basic feeling of being him.

to communicate in a foreign language. I realized how much **looser, freer, and more flowing I am** in my body gestures than he is."

—SANDY, AGE 26

The aim of the role-playing game is to spread understanding and not to be hurtful. If something negative comes to mind, resist acting on it; create harmony, not humiliation. After this short, fifteen-minute introduction to role-playing your partner, you may wish to extend this game for an hour some other evening, enacting the first time you met, or even choose to go to bed in your opposite roles.

GET INTO CHARACTER

Dressed in each other's robes, come into the Sensual Space embodied as the other person. Hug, gaze at each other, and kiss one another. Light the candles, and prepare the space, moving through the room in the style of your partner. Sit down opposite one another and decide who will give the first Weather Report. Who usually does what in determining this opening step between you? Set the timer for two minutes (who usually does it?). In your Weather Report, talk using the voice and mannerisms of your partner, and choose the subject matter as he would. If you're brave, try a Come Clean!

Clear negative space as well as call in positive energy in the style he typically does. Gesture like he would. Set an intention similarly worded to the ones you've heard your partner speak before. End the Opening Ritual by exchanging with your partner a two-minute-each Body Caress or massage of your choice. In character, figure out who gets what first, and then caress or massage in the style of your partner's touch. End with a Heart Salutation, and switch back to own robe and role without talking about the exercise.

Erotic Exercise 2: **Playing the Yin/Yang Game**   [SEVENTY-FIVE MINUTES EACH]

To play the Yin/Yang Game, you have to first know how to play Yang and play Yin.

PLAYING YANG

When playing Yang in this consensual exercise, do not be afraid to use power. You often see so much misuse of power around you that you might fear all power is aggressive and violent. Anchor yourself in the use of positive power, the power to come from love, the power to oversee, protect, and care for those servants in your care. Full-bodied power is reverent toward your submitter and expresses appreciation for his service and gifts. Positive power moves you to dare, invent, command, and make your fantasies come true.

Use your powerful position to better understand your desires, expand your erotic imagination, and initiate and lead confidently in the relationship. The container of your trusting and honest intimate partnership will provide a safe haven in which to explore forgotten or feared parts of yourself. Empower yourself with love to gain greater self-knowledge. Play this game with the wild spirit of a child and the caring consciousness of an adult.

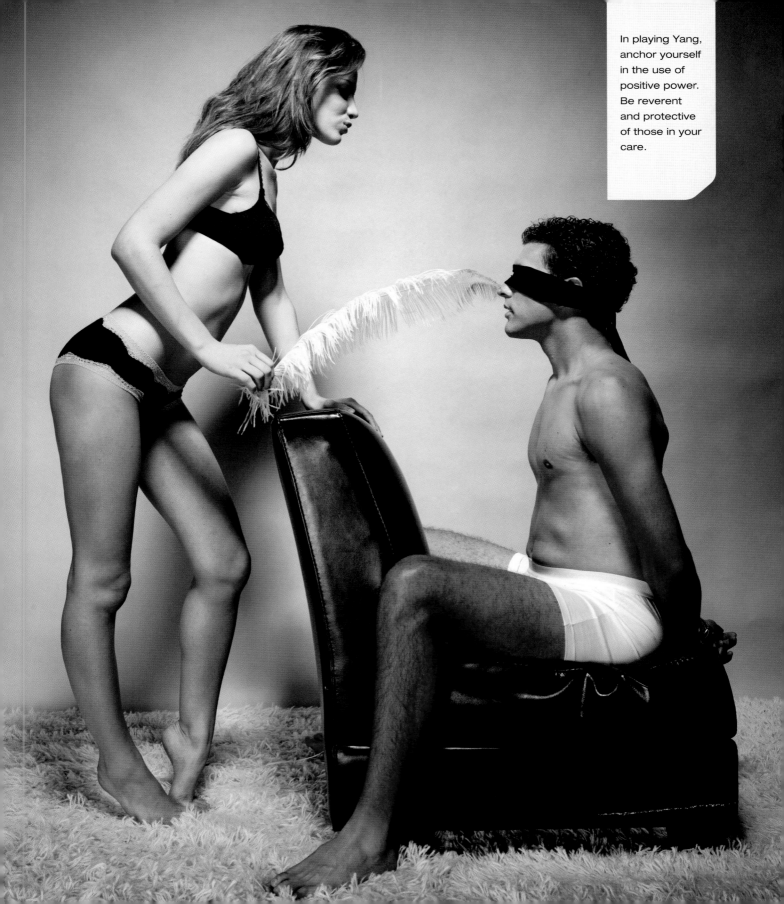

In playing Yang, anchor yourself in the use of positive power. Be reverent and protective of those in your care.

PLAYING YIN

As you explore the surrendering role of Yin, you submit because you consciously negoti-ated this role for your personal growth and pleasure. You submit because you want to, not because you have to. As the serving partner, you acknowledge at all times the integrity of your boundaries and the ability to say yes or no. At the same time, you seek to expand your boundaries and exercise your yes-saying to things that may stretch you or be unfamiliar.

As Yin, you learn to soften your ego and let go of the need to do things your way. You melt your hard edges to flow into the greater whole, experiencing the peace and joy of sur-render. In conscious power exchanges, you voluntarily lose yourself in service to another so that you may reclaim hidden parts of yourself and expand your erotic palette. You choose submission in the context of a safe and responsible relationship knowing you picked a Yang partner whom you can.

PLAYING THE GAME

Choose who will be Yang first, and set the timer for seventy-five minutes. Do you have a special appellation that you'd like to be addressed as, like Majesty Queen, Wizard Master, Boss, or Your Highness? Do you have a special costume or pet name for your serving Yin partner? When you are Yang and tire of or are not pleased by the status quo, tweak it. Choose another activity from your list, or make up something new in the moment. Be a spontaneous tyrant to your demands. Be present to your wishes as they arise moment to moment and express them. You're the boss.

If a beloved is not dancing sexily enough, command her to gyrate her hips this way or that. Tell her to wet her lips and blow you kisses. If an original love poem isn't gushy enough, have your partner go down on his or her knees, look up at you lovingly like a puppy and pant as he counts even more ways he loves you. Do not humiliate your servant; rather, reward your beloved copiously for his or her performance. Make sure any massages and caresses are just the way you like them, and do not compromise. This is your night in heaven, and your angel is there to make it perfect. Keep your standards high, and lavish your approval.

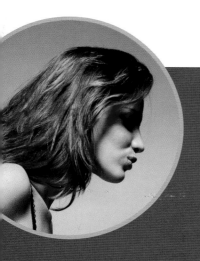

"I was receiving a 'too soft' massage from my Yang partner. Never before had I been able to tell him to use more pressure. Then I thought, 'Hey, I'm Yang. **If I can't ask for what I what**

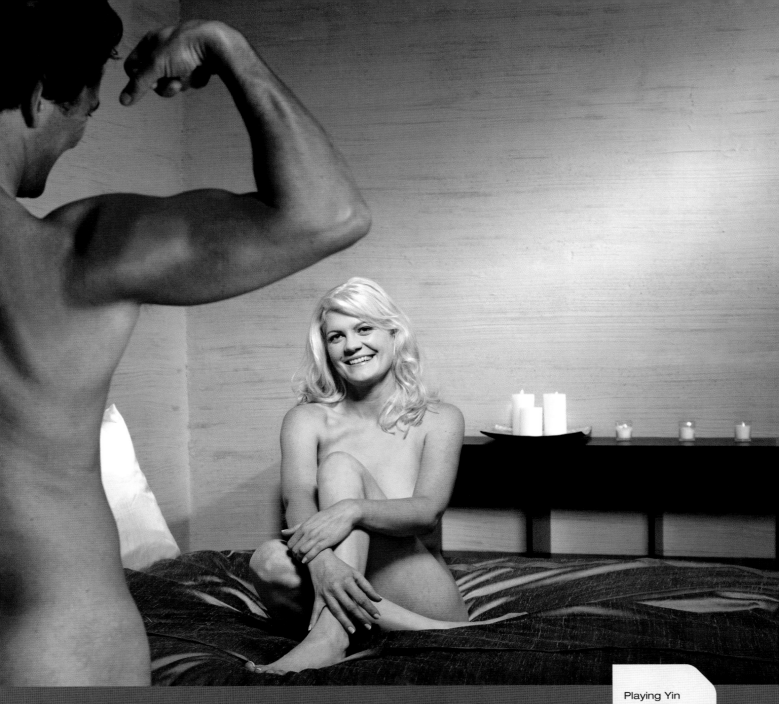

now, when can I?' I blurted it out, and it felt liberating to ask for it how I liked it. It broke the ice of him thinking that he has to be perfect and know everything. **This game will help our sex life!"**

—PAULA, AGE 45

Playing Yin softens the ego and the need to do things your way. You serve and surrender.

As the Yin partner, if you receive a request that is not to your liking, try saying something like, "Dearest King, I regret that I cannot fulfill that request. But I so wish to please my master—what other wish may I have the pleasure to serve you with?" The final say always lies with the Yin person, because doing anything disagreeable to your pleasure violates the number one rule of great sex: "Do what brings you pleasure."

At the end of seventy-five minutes, stand before one another and share a Heart Salutation as a way of honoring the divine feminine and masculine at play in each of us. Feel the pleasure that conscious play brings to your partnership. Shake off your role literally with a full-body shake. Reset the timer, and switch roles for the next seventy-five minutes.

PLAY THE YIN/YANG GAME FOR A WEEKEND

I first learned of the Yin/Yang Game from reading Margot Anand's *The Art of Sexual Ecstasy.* One of my most erotic weekends ever was when my beloved and I played the Yin/Yang Game for forty-eight hours over a weekend. Every moment is etched in my memory, from waking up and being served breakfast, to long massages naked on the patio, to a blindfolded walk in the park, to being treated to dinner with the rule of talking only in three-word sentences, to being bathed and sung to that night. The next day, being Yin was equally riveting. My beloved wanted me to be his slave girl and commanded me to walk ahead of him at the farmer's market while shopping. I couldn't look at him or react when he touched me. I obeyed his every demand at the market, and then he ordered me to carry the picnic basket to our secluded spot and answer "Yes, Master" to all his commands. I could hardly contain my excitement.

Erotic Exercise 3: Closing Ritual [TEN MINUTES]

Tonight you role-played your partner to better understand how gender colors how you speak and move in the world. You played consciously with power and surrender dynamics in the Yin/Yang Game to awaken greater potential to direct and follow in erotic scenarios.

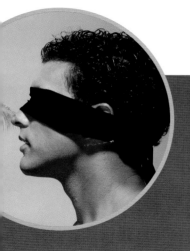

"Playing the Yin/Yang Game was delicious. I stepped back from the initiator role and watched her lead the juicy show . . . her way. I was a glutton for surrender to her every desire.

In closing, sit opposite one another, and set the timer for five minutes. Take turns talking about your experience role-playing your partner and playing the Yin/Yang Game. Listen for essence without adding your comments, and ask a question only if you need to clarify what your partner is saying. At the end of five minutes, exchange roles. Here are some questions you may wish to include in your sharing:

- What did I learn about myself seeing my partner role-play me?
- What did I learn about the opposite gender by role-playing my partner?
- What was the most difficult/fulfilling part of the Yin/Yang Game for me?
- Did I really ask for what I wanted when I was Yang, or did I compromise?
- Could I really surrender as Yin and feel safe? What was playing Yin like for me?
- Would I like to play this game for a longer time frame, such as a long weekend?

Looking Ahead

- Write four lists in your Ecstasy Journal under the following topics: What turns me on sexually? What would I never do sexually? What do I fantasize about sexually? And what would I like to try sexually but have not yet?
- Read Erotic Night Eight several days before it takes place.

Erotic Recap

- Preparing for the Yin/Yang Game
- Opening Ritual: *fifteen minutes*
- Playing the Yin/Yang Game: *seventy-five minutes each*
- Closing Ritual: *ten minutes*

The time was over too soon. I want to play the Yin/Yang Game for **a whole heavenly weekend.**"

—RICHARD, AGE 34

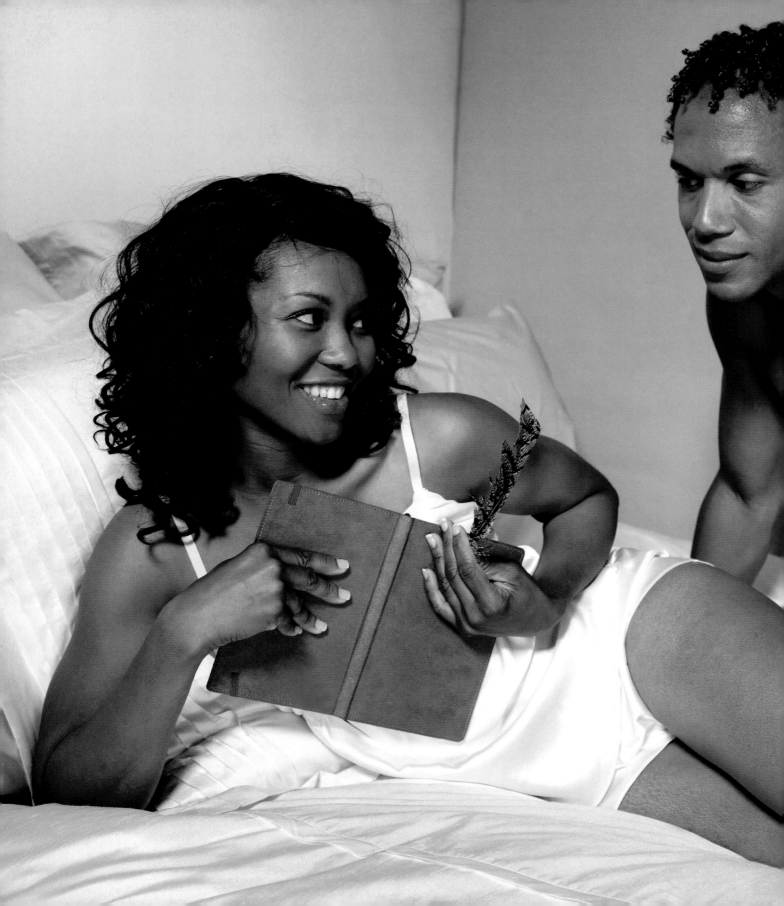

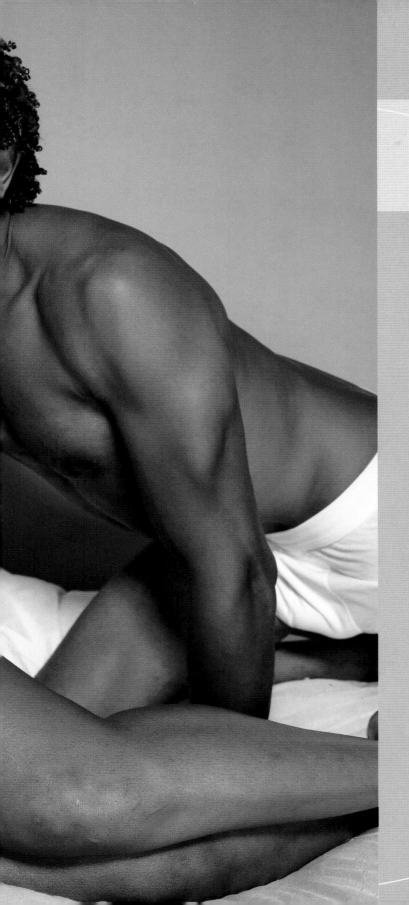

EROTIC NIGHT
EIGHT

Addressing
Challenging
Issues and
Charging Your
Sexuality

EROTIC NIGHT EIGHT

During the previous Erotic Night, you role-played the opposite gender, experienced power and surrender dynamics in the Yin/Yang Game, and practiced how to ask for and offer deep erotic gifts. On your last Erotic Night, you will learn ways to discuss challenging sexual issues and charge your sexuality by uncovering your sexual shadow and fantasies.

Bring your Ecstasy Journal, complete with your four lists: (1) sexual turn-ons, (2) sexual-never-will-do's, (3) sexual fantasies, and (4) what-I-want-to-do-sexually-but-haven't-yets. Show up on time with a full heart, focused mind, and relaxed and energized body, ready to be present with your partner.

Erotic Exercise 1: Opening Ritual   [TWENTY MINUTES]

With the sacred attitude befitting the Priest and Priestess of Pleasure you are becoming, light your candles, and prepare your Sensual Space for this last Erotic Night. Sit opposite one another, and set the timer for your Weather Reports. Can you appreciate this concise, respectful format to routinely check in with one another? Keeping within the time frames keeps this ritual powerful and interesting.

By releasing negativity and affirming the positive all within a few seconds, you can turn your evening from ordinary to sacred. Offer a short sentence of release and intention. Within a half minute, you can construct an intentional reality, such as, "I release my tensions of the day, and I call into my evening a golden light of love." State your intention in one breath, such as, "I intend to grow love in my family and partnership." You don't get two breaths; the truth is simple.

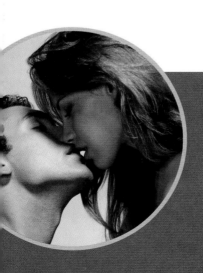

"The Tantric Kiss helps me **prolong my arousal.** The waves of orgasmic pleasure come and go, and I don't even have to act on them. **I've realized my power as a lover.** I can hold the container for the magic between us."

—DAVID, AGE 49

OCEAN BREATHE WITH SPINAL MOVEMENT

You have practiced the ancient and erotic Tantric Kiss, in which you learned to slow your breathing, include pauses at the top and bottom of the breath, and add PC Pulses during the pauses. You have learned alternate breathing, in which one partner is breathing in while the other is breathing out. The final piece of this sacred erotic ritual is moving the spine with the breath. Then the Tantric Kiss, an exchange of divine essences with your partner, is complete. Take a breath mint before continuing.

If you've ever watched a newborn baby, you'll see that her whole spine moves with each inhale and exhale. Movement is an important way to build erotic energy in the body. Do you remember finding the pleasure of repetitive movement when you were a child? It was probably by accident. Perhaps you were playing on the teeter-totter, sitting on a log, or even sitting on a parent's lap, and you started rocking into a euphoric trance, although you didn't have the name for it yet.

To practice moving the spine with the breath, both partners get on their hands and knees on the floor and begin deep, slow-sounding Ocean Breathing. As you breathe out, arch your back up to the ceiling pulling, your belly button up toward your spine with your head moving toward the floor. As you breathe in, arch your back in the opposite direction,

Spinal movement helps build erotic excitement in the body.

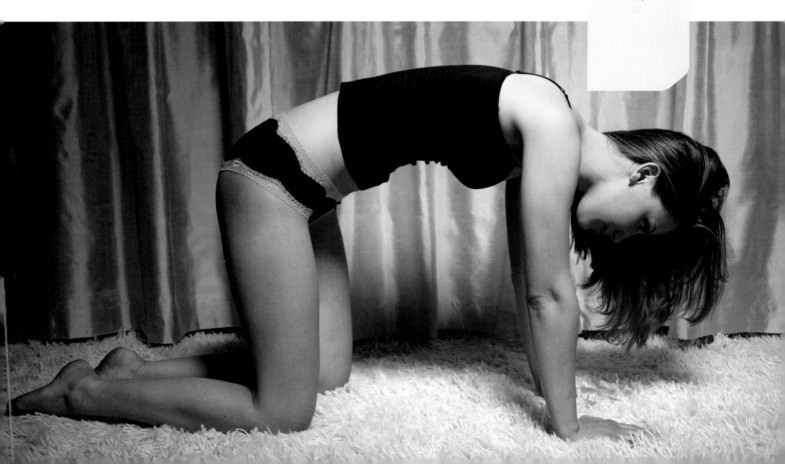

toward the floor, and lift your head and butt toward the ceiling. Keep your belly soft. Repeat for several minutes, exaggerating this movement. Flexing the spine in this way also prepares the body for greater ease and freedom in sex.

Now try this spinal movement in a sitting position. Sit opposite each other in a loose yab-yum position, the woman's legs over the man's thighs. Using the same spinal movement as when you were on all fours, exhale together, curving the spine into a C-shape, head forward, and inhale, letting the pelvis fall forward (soft belly) and head back. If you are not already pausing at the top and bottom of the breath, do so now. Once established, the man inverts his breath and breaths out when his partner breathes in for Alternate Sexual Breathing with Spinal Movement.

Deepen your connection to one another through Alternate Sexual Breathing in the yab-yum position.

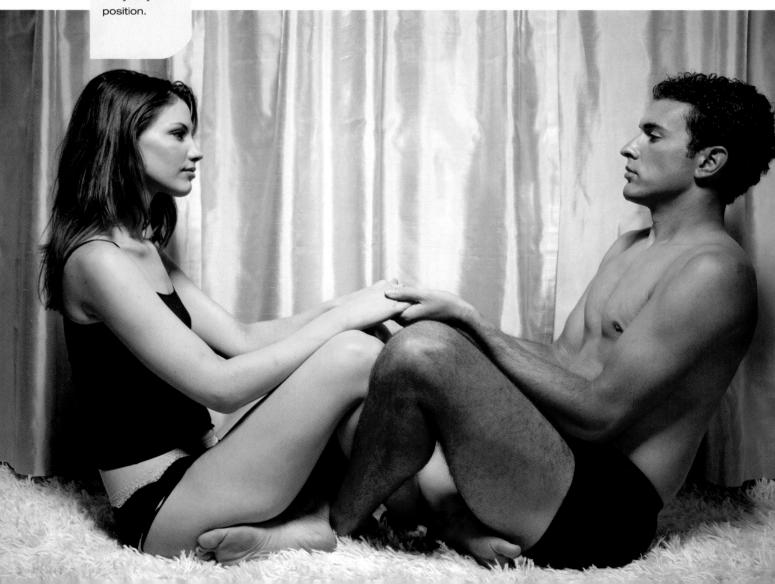

Set the timer for five minutes and have the woman sit in the man's lap in yab-yum position, her head above his. Loosely kiss so as not to form suction. Continue with the Alternate Sexual Breathing with Spinal Movement. Feel the movement of your bodies together. Add PC Pulses—especially long, slow squeezes—when you are inspired. On the exhale, the woman visualizes her love going into her partner's heart, and on the inhale receiving his love up through her *yoni* (vagina). On the inhale, the man visualizes taking the woman's love into his heart, and on the exhale he send his love into her *yoni* through his *lingam* (penis).

Feel yourself as the source of your pleasure. Feel the eternal circle of love and goodwill between you and your partner. You are balancing and gifting each other with each breath. It's okay if you get lost, just pick it up the best you can. Enjoy this treasured and timeless way to weave weightlessly in and out of each other. Allow your bodies to merge, dissolve, reappear, and float in a loving, formless sea of being. Erotic trance heals and rejuvenates the body; allow it to wash over you. See in your beloved's eyes the youthful, relaxed, and energized look of erotic trance states.

Erotic Exercise 2: **Addressing Challenging Sexual Issues by Agreement**   [THIRTY MINUTES]

In my sex coaching practice, I find the most damaging aspect of any sexual relationship between couples is the secrecy of their sex lives and withholding sexual truths from one another. Similar to what you learned in Coming Clean, it's what is not said that can hurt you. Most couples do not openly talk about sex. They especially don't discuss how to make honest and honorable agreements about the difficult sexual issues in their relationship.

Without talking, and often in the midst of misery, you may each assume you have some kind of ownership and control over your partner's sex life. It's easy to assume that you can expect your partner to exclude everyone else but you in sexual activity—even if you are sexually bored, inactive, unavailable, medically impaired, or actively flirting or being sexual with others.

Silence and secrecy, as well as assuming ownership of a partner's sexuality, causes depression, infidelity, anxiety, and breakdown (divorce) in many couples. Not only does sexual secrecy and controlling behaviors make both partners miserable, it deeply damages people with feelings of guilt, shame, and jealousy. These emotions are life-sucking and health-threatening. Somehow, society has turned jealousy into a normal, even good, emotion, leading one to believe, "If s/he gets jealous of my other interests, then it means s/he loves me." Jealousy, or needing to control another's life, is a product of low self-esteem, insecurity, and fear of abandonment. It is a natural feeling only in a society that allows self-destructive and damaging emotions to be regarded as normal.

WHAT IS SEX?

In conventional monogamous relationships, the benchmark is to be nonsexual with everyone but your partner. But what does that mean? The word sex, like the word love, can be very small or very large. You love pizza and you love your mother. If sex is defined solely as the penis-in-the-vagina or the penetration of genitals (skin-to-skin, wiggle-wiggle, pop orgasm), that is one thing. If sex is to have a larger meaning, which includes the multitude of erotic impulses, imagination, fantasies, desires, and attractions that are inherent in our moment-to-moment life, then sex is another thing and not so circumscribed—or controllable. Someone may choose to have genital penetration with only one partner, exclusively, until death but not be able to stop thoughts and imagination of sexual activities with others. In the larger definition of sex, there is no such thing as sexual exclusivity.

It's in this larger definition of sex or eroticism (sexual love) that life becomes more chaotic, wildly individual, and difficult to manage neatly. We are all unique sexual snowflakes, and not all of us fit tidily into one standard box—unless we let others beat us into the box with a heavy hand of guilt, dogma, shame, and ignorance. We are all unique mosaics of past sexual experiences, obstacles, and attractions that makes any coupling "doubly unique" and relationships doubly impossible to fit into a one-size-fits-all model.

You can't take the erotic out of a human being. When your partner is or is not around, you are still a sexual being with imagination, desires, and attractions. When you acknowledge eroticism as an inherent, pervasive, and natural part of human nature that percolates within you, you're in a good position to deal creatively and positively with your own sexuality and the challenges of authentic relationship sex. Further, when you choose to recognize eroticism as a graceful and beautiful part of being human, you are in a good position to have rapturous sex and be honest about it.

MAKE SEXUAL AGREEMENTS WITH YOUR PARTNER

As a couple, you can create your own "box" of agreements of erotic do's and don'ts that work for you—and agree to change what's in the box whenever you want. Your container can grow and take shape as you grow. Instead of the old model, run by silence, unrealistic expectations, ownership, hiding, and lying, you can craft a new model. You can make changeable agreements with your partner over challenging sexual issues that encourage integrity and openness.

Savvy couples who engage in responsible sexual conversations win the respect and attention of each other, over and over. As healthy, naturally sexy beings at large in the world, we yearn to stay excitably alive and authentic in our interactions with others and at the same time honor our commitments to our valued partnership.

To do that, engage in frequent conversations about sexual matters, and air your needs and fears so you may agree together on what is and is not permissible at this point in your relationship. Write down your agreements, and sign them as a matter of record. Revisit your agreements whenever either of you no longer chooses to abide by them. When you violates your agreement, you need to tell your partner and apologize. Agreements are living documents that can be amended.

Challenging issues you and your partner can come to agreement on include the following.

- **One partner wants intercourse or wants sensual touching more often than the other.** What are creative ways to handle differences in desire for touching? Can you ask for more cuddle time and put a time frame on it? Can you hold your lover while s/he

You can make changeable sexual agreements with your partner on sexual issues that encourage integrity and openness.

Self-Pleasures if you're not interested in intercourse? Can nongenital massage and caress be part of your regular exchanges in your relationship? Can you go outside of the relationship for this touch? Is massage with genital touching part of the relationship? Is it okay outside of the relationship? What about orgasmic release with massage? Are intercourse or oral sex with sex professionals options?

•   **The amount of time that is desirable for foreplay, intercourse, and aftercare.** Are "quickies" okay? How often? Does each partner get enough long, languorous, prolonged intimate play? Time of day, place, and other variables may be topics for discussion and agreement.

•   **Sexual exploration.** Discuss and make agreements on viewing sex education, Tantra, or pornographic movies together. You may agree to explore together, alone, or not at all on the Internet, in chat rooms, with erotica literature, through phone sex, or with anal touching/or sex. You may also explore bondage-discipline-sadomasochistic activities in intentional communities.

•   **Attractions to other people and fantasies with others.** Is talking about your attractions and fantasies about others an erotic turn-on for you or your partner? Do you prefer not to share that information?

•   **Genital penetration with someone besides your partner.** Your response may be a resounding no to this issue. However, if there's negotiating room, under what safe-sex conditions is it permitted? Do new play partners need prior approval by your primary partner? Are location and timing important? What other considerations need to be agreed upon for the safe and respectful handling of this sensitive issue? A book like *The Ethical Slut* by Dossie Easton and Catherine A. Liszt is a good reference to design responsible polyamorous relationships.

•   **Nonpenetration sexual play with someone besides your partner.** This also may be a flat no. If it's a maybe or yes, what activities are okay? Flirting, kissing, nongenital touching, petting with genital touching, oral sex? Under what conditions would any of the above be okay. . . with people you know, don't know, with or without permission of the primary partner, in locations outside your hometown, etc.? Do you choose to talk about experiences with other lovers as a couple?

•   **Involving other people in partnership sexual play.** You may want to discuss and make agreements on having other people join you and your partner for different kinds of sensual or sexual play. You and your partner may agree to having sex in the presence of others such as at sex clubs or parties.

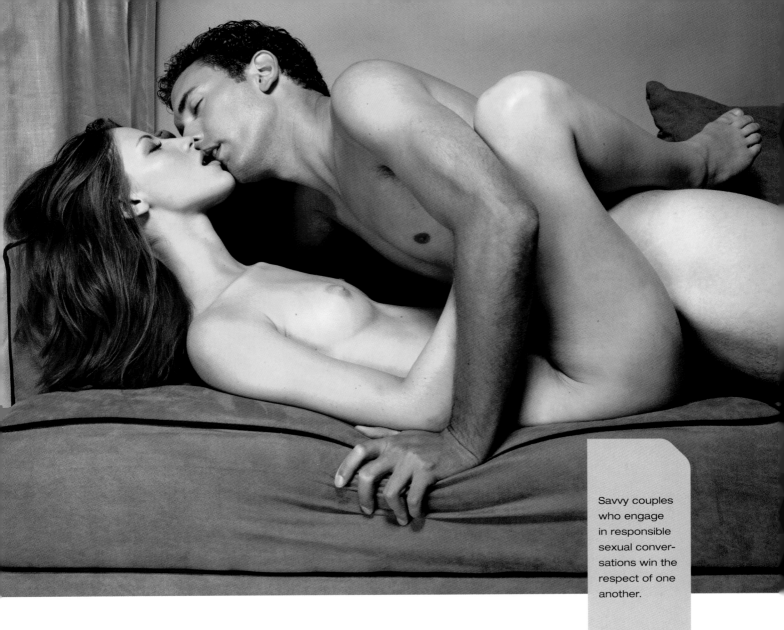

COMMIT TO MAKING SEXUAL AGREEMENTS WITH YOUR PARTNER

In your Ecstasy Journals, make a page for Sexual Agreements with your partner. Write down a few things that are on your mind that you may like to discuss together for possible Sexual Agreements at a later date. Decide on a date to make Sexual Agreements and address challenging issues in your partnership. Write the meeting date and time on your calendars, and remember, Sexual Agreements work best if they are written down, dated, and initialed; they can always be changed.

Erotic Exercise 3: **Charging Your Sexuality** [FIFTEEN MINUTES]

If you are reading this chapter in preparation for the last Erotic Night, do not read this section, because it will ruin the surprise at the end. Leave this exercise to be done on the spot on the last Erotic Night and begin instead to read the next section on sexual turn-ons.

This is a fun exercise to help you learn more about yourself and to bring new strengths into your sexual relationship.

1. **Describe who you are.** Set the timer for three minutes, and open to a new page in your Ecstasy Journals. Draw a circle that fills almost the entire page, and draw a horizontal line dividing the circle in half. On the top half of the circle, write down many personality traits that describe you—the things you identify as being you. Write down words that describe how you see yourself, such as, "handsome, reserved, humorous, efficient, serious, successful, polite, hard worker, clean, etc." Write intuitively, without thinking too much about it. Keep your pen moving as much of the time as possible. Come up with at least ten personality traits that describe you.

2. **Describe who you are not.** After you have finished with the words that best describe or identify you on the top half of your circle, reset the timer for three minutes and, in the bottom half, write all the personality traits that you do not identify with. Write all the things that you are not. These words may describe how others are, but not you. Begin writing all the things that you do not identify as being you for the next three minutes.

3. **Share these qualities.** After you have finished the lower half of your circle, the person with the darkest eyes will begin by sharing the qualities on the top half only of her list. Read to your partner all the ways in which you see yourself, the things you are, and the traits you identify with. Do not comment while your partner is reading her list; simply listen. Now switch, and have the other partner read the list of traits he believes describes him. After you both have disclosed your self-images, take turns sharing the words on the bottom of the circle, those with which you do NOT identify. This should take between five and ten minutes.

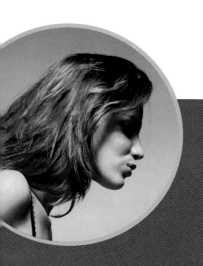

"I about died and got wet in my pants when I discovered my boyfriend's lower circle—**dominating, being tyrannical, and manipulating**

4. **Conclude the exercise.** When you have completed this exercise, give each other a Heart Salutation. The interesting thing about this exercise is that what charges or expands your sexual arena generally comes from the traits in the bottom half of the circle rather than those in the top half. In other words, that which you resist being, or resist identifying with, or have not yet fully integrated into your personality, is often your greatest gift to expand sexual play.

The traits from the bottom half of the circle are attributes that you have yet to embrace into your life and sex life. You may even think these traits are improper, which, interestingly enough, can be the antidote to sexual routine and boredom. What you push away or have yet to embrace into your sex lives can spark sexual growth and discovery. Take a look at your list from that standpoint, have a laugh, and talk with your partner about how you may invite those qualities into your sex life for fun.

Erotic Exercise 4: Turn-ons, Never-Will-Do's, Fantasies, and What-I-Want-to-Do-but-Haven't-Yet [TWENTY MINUTES]

Keep your Ecstasy Journals out for yet another exercise to further explore your sexuality with your partner. Review the four lists you brought as homework to this evening. Journal assignments are for you and are confidential, so if you choose not to share from your lists, you may skip this section. No judgments. Or you may choose to share one or more items (or all) from each category as a way to increase sexual enlightenment and opportunity.

Finding out what turns your partner on and off, understanding your partner's sexual imagination, and learning about the things your partner would like to try sexually but has not yet is important intimate geography to cover, if not tonight, then at some point soon. If tonight is the night:

1. **Decide who will go first, start with the first category, and read from your list of sexual turn-ons as much as you are willing to share.**

others. I thought, hot! I was charged! When can we start playing? He was confused, but I helped him figure it out."

—TERESA, AGE 55

2. **Exchange roles listening and speaking.** For the next three categories, change who starts first. Do not comment or judge; rather, thank your partner after each sharing.

It feels vulnerable to disclose sexual information that you have been conditioned to believe is private (or shameful). However, you are not private about your favorite foods, hobbies, people, music, or movies. Why has sex become so hidden, if not for shame? Here's your chance to undo the limits of shame. Let it out. Give yourself permission to be the outrageously weird, sassy, kinky, and one-of-a-kind sexual creature that you are. Give voice to your unique sexual landscape. Celebrate your unique path and journey. Share things about what you want and have not experienced. You are building truth with your partner. Open your hearts to the place of nonjudgment. When you love yourself, you can truly love your partner.

Erotic Exercise 5: Acting Out a Fantasy or a Haven't-Done-Yet [SEVENTY MINUTES]

After the rich sharing of your journal lists, select a fantasy or a yet-to-do experience that you can ask your partner to help make come true. Keep the conversation open until you find one that pleases you both. This act of courage and truth is a celebration of the trust you have built with your partner in your Eight Erotic Nights together. You are sexual pioneers. You showed up for pleasure, paid attention, told the truth, and expressed your desires. You crafted a clear and clean container for sexual rapture by appreciating, honoring, healing, and playing with your partner.

You each have thirty-five minutes to design your play on this last night of the series. You have the tools to express your desires and do what pleases you, to say yes and no, and to respect the other's no. Use these tools to find your common denominator for pleasure with your partner. What will it be? Set the timer for thirty-five minutes, and explore new sexual territory or, if you'd rather, repeat any exercises in this book.

"My lover and I exchanged our lists over the phone, and I think it worked great. It made it easier for me, and we didn't have to act on anything right away. **I feel I know him so much better now.**"

—TANYA, AGE 25

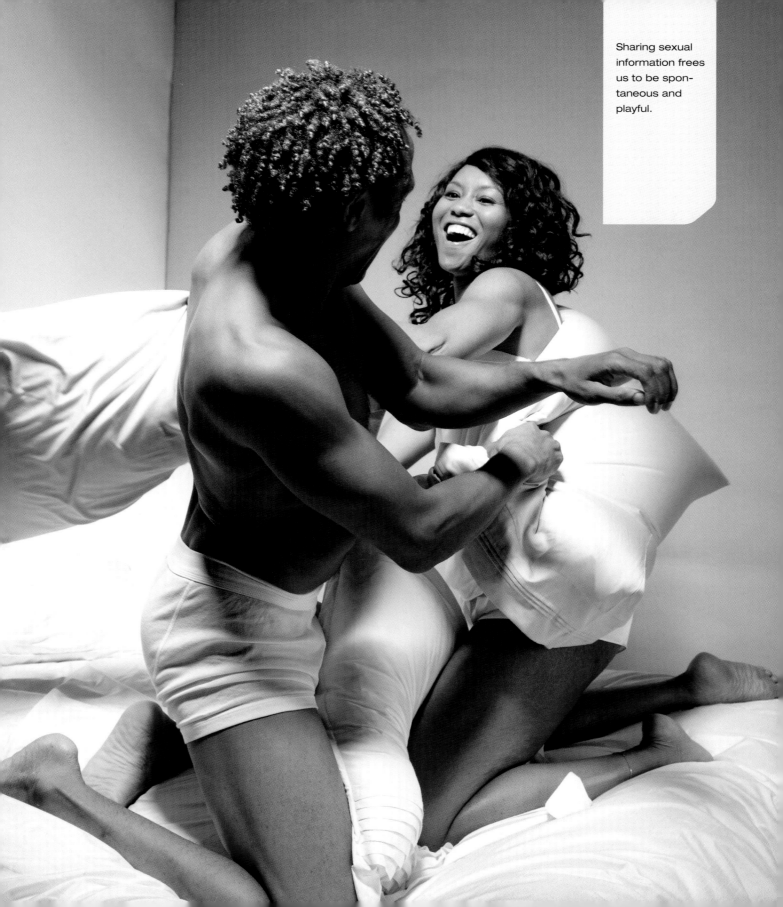

Sharing sexual
information frees
us to be spon-
taneous and
playful.

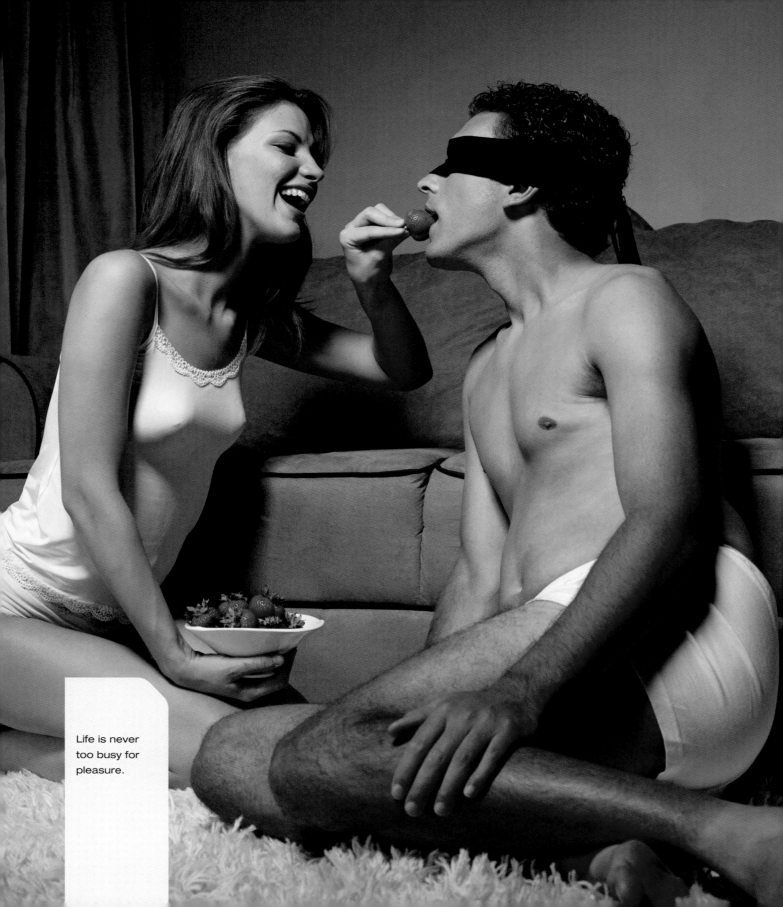

Life is never
too busy for
pleasure.

If you need a toy, props, or special clothes for your fantasy, plan when you will do this, and make your own date for playing out the fantasy. Upon completion of *Eight Erotic Nights,* you will be in charge of scheduling your own date nights and making room for pleasure in your busy lives. How will that look? What commitments are you willing to make? Write them down in your Ecstasy Journals.

Upon completion of both play sessions, remember that what is spoken and acted out in your Sensual Space stays there. You may revisit tonight's activities only by receiving permission from your partner. You are creating a trusting vessel. Be proud of crafting a sexually alive and authentic relationship. When you make mistakes, tell you partner, apologize, and ask for forgiveness. In the safety of confidentiality, you can be the fool, make mistakes, play in the bottom half of the circle, and claim the great sex you were born—wired, really—to enjoy.

Erotic Exercise 6: Closing Ritual [TWENTY MINUTES]

In closing, sit opposite one another. The partner who will be active first sets the timer for four minutes. Talk about what you do not like about yourself and what you do not want others to know about you. Share a Heart Salutation, and trade roles.

For the final round set, take turns telling each other what you do like about yourself for another four minutes. After each of you speaks, receive from your partner a two-minute Face Caress. Bow in gratitude to one another. Perform your closing gesture, blow out the candles, and leave your Sensual Space. You carry with you the tools to create anew at anytime, anywhere, with anybody a conscious, intentional environment for discovery. Sense yourself as the source of your own rapture.

Erotic Recap

- Opening Ritual: *twenty minutes*
- Addressing Challenging Sexual Issues by Agreement: *thirty minutes*
- Charging Your Sexuality: *fifteen minutes*
- Turn-ons, Never-Will-Do's, Fantasies, and What-I-Want-to-Do-but-Haven't-Yet: *twenty minutes*
- Acting Out a Fantasy or a Haven't-Done-Yet: *seventy minutes*
- Closing Ritual: *twenty minutes*

Acknowledgments

As an intimacy coach, I thank every man, woman, and couple who has ever showed up at my door longing to connect with the heart, soul, and spirit of their loving. I acknowledge you as Seekers, as my teachers, often my peers, none of you dysfunctional, and all of you whole and capable of profound loving. I bow to you and every Pilgrim of Ecstasy who has ever risked being totally authentic in sexual exploration. You hold up the mirror to my challenges, my fears, and my joys of becoming an amazing lover.

I thank you, rebellious reader, for choosing this book as a pathway to ecstasy and passion. You choose sacred embodiment over shame, truth over silence, and freedom over the mundane. You manifest the new paradigm for erotic grace and truth defined by acceptance, appreciation, openness, and respect.

I pay tribute to my teachers of erotic wellness who have touched me deeply with their wisdom. I thank Joseph Kramer, courageous leader in positive sex education (eroticmassage.com); Barnaby B. Barratt, author of *Sexual Health and Erotic Freedom*; Reid Mihalko and Marcia Baczynski, founders of Cuddle Party (cuddleparty.com); Antra and Richard Borofsky, workshop facilitators on intimacy (beingtogether.com); Betty Martin, erotic educator for touch professionals (eroticeducation.org); Marshall Rosenberg (nonviolent-communication.com); Linda Poelzl, president of the Association of Certified Sexological Bodyworkers (sexologicalbodywork.com); and Alex Jade, teacher of power and surrender in intimacy.

I thank my courageous family for being pioneers each in their own way. I am grateful for each and every person who has ever touched me, however casual or profound, for showing me another aspect of my own journey and growth towards becoming Love. And I thank Stephen, whose profound attention, passion, and insight helped me test-drive and fine-tune this book's eight erotic nights…with joy.

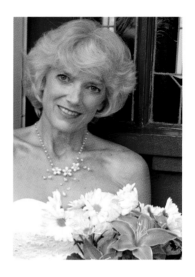

About the Author

Charla Hathaway is the founder of BodyJoy, a school for the erotic arts in Austin, Texas. She coaches couples in sex and intimacy, and leads erotic-spiritual play for men and women in classes, workshops, and retreats.

Author of *Erotic Massage: Sensual Touch for Deep Pleasure and Extended Arousal,* Charla is also a certified sexological body-worker, Sacred Intimate, Tantra teacher, and founding member of the Association of Sexual Energy Professionals. Teaching sacred embodiment is her passion and joy. Visit her at www.bodyjoy.org.